OVERVIEW
OF
OCULAR
DISORDERS

OVERVIEW OF OCULAR DISORDERS

Nancy T. Gwin, FCLSA, COT
Director of Contact Lens Services
Premier Medical Eye Group
Mobile, Alabama

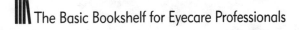 The Basic Bookshelf for Eyecare Professionals

Series Editors: Janice K. Ledford, COMT • Ken Daniels, OD • Robert Campbell, MD

SLACK INCORPORATED 6900 Grove Road, Thorofare, NJ 08086

Publisher: John H. Bond
Editorial Director: Amy E. Drummond
Assistant Editor: Lauren Biddle

Correct ISBN for
Overview of Ocular Disorders
by Nancy Gwin is 1-55642-336-5

Gwin, Nancy T.
    Overview of Ocular Disorders/ Nancy T. Gwin
        p. cm. — (The basic bookshelf for eyecare professionals)
        Includes bibliographical references and index.
        ISBN 1-55642-334-9 (alk. paper)
        1. Eye—Diseases. I. Title. II. Series.
        [DNLM: 1. Eye diseases. 2. Eyelid diseases. 3. Vision disorders
    WW 140 G994o 1998]
    RE46.G95 1998
    617.7'1—DC21
    DNLM/DLC
    for Library of Congress   98-43416
                                                                  CIP

Published by: SLACK Incorporated
                  6900 Grove Road
                  Thorofare, NJ 08086-9447 USA
                  Telephone: 609-848-1000
                  Fax: 609-853-5991
                  World Wide Web: http://www.slackinc.com

Last digit is print number: 10   9   8   7   6   5   4   3   2   1

Dedication

For my parents, Perry and Syble Thomas, who always encouraged and loved me.

Contents

Acknowledgments

Special thanks to my cousin and friend, Gloria Roskoski, for all the hours of typing; and to Jan Ledford, my editor, for all the direction and editing during the writing process of this book.

About the Author

Nancy Thomas Gwin began working in ophthalmology in 1971 for Premier Medical Eye Group, Mobile, Alabama, where she is now Director of Contact Lens Services. In addition to her duties as director, she fits specialty contact lenses.

Ms. Gwin is NCLE Certified as well as a Certified Ophthalmic Technician (COT). She is a Fellow in the Contact Lens Society of America, serving on their Board of Directors and as editor of their quarterly publication, the *EyeWitness*. She is also a member of Contact Lens Association of Ophthalmologists (CLAO) and the Opticians Association of America (OAA).

Her passions are challenging contact lens fits and traveling.

Introduction

This book is a basic overview of disorders of the eye. Its purpose is to "get you started." Successfully recognizing ocular problems is an on-going learning process. Ask mentors and fellow workers to share their interesting cases with you. Patients almost always give their permission to allow other technicians to observe pathology. They seem to enjoy being part of the education process.

It is important for the reader of this book – one who wants to be more knowledgeable about recognizing complications – to take responsibility. Do not wait for others to show you; ask to see everything!

Good luck in your quest to become more familiar with ocular complications. Let this book be just the beginning.

A Note About Patient Education: Most books in the Basic Bookshelf series have boxed-in material (sidebars) containing patient education information. Because every section in *Ocular Disorders* could conceivably have such sidebars, we have elected not to use the sidebar in this book. However, the information in any section, if put into terms that the layman can understand, may be used to educate the patient about his or her disease process, its treatment and prognosis.

Nancy T. Gwin, FCLSA, COT

The Study Icons

The *Basic Bookshelf for Eyecare Professionals* is quality educational material designed for professionals in all branches of eyecare. Because so many of you want to expand your careers, we have made a special effort to include information needed for certification exams. When these study icons appear in the margin of a *Series* book, it is your cue that the material next to the icon (which may be a paragraph or an entire section) is listed as a criteria item for a certification examination. Please use this key to identify the appropriate icon:

OptA   optometric assistant

OptT   optometric technician

OphA   ophthalmic assistant

OphT   ophthalmic technician

OphMT   ophthalmic medical technologist

LV   low vision subspecialty

Srg   ophthalmic surgical assisting subspecialty

CL   contact lens registry*

Optn   opticianry*

RA   retinal angiographer

*Note: The certification criteria for these specialties are ambiguous regarding oular disease, simply stating "pathology" or eye conditions." While this book is useful for all listed specialties, we have not attempted to code the text for these two areas.

Chapter 1

Skin and Eyelids

KEY POINTS

- Any disorder that results in lashes contacting the globe can cause corneal damage.

- It is important to have any suspicious growth of the skin and eyelids checked by a physician.

- During a biopsy, tissue is removed, fixed in a 40% formaldehyde solution, and sent to a laboratory for analysis.

- Blepharitis is the most common inflammation of the eyelids and is often associated with conjunctivitis and dry eye syndrome.

Abnormalities/Disorders/Anomalies/Growths

Entropion

Entropion is an inward-turning of the eyelid, usually the lower, so that the lid margin brushes against the eyeball (Figure 1-1). It is more common in elderly people who have lost muscle and skin tone. Entropion is functionally important because the inward-turning lashes may cause damage to the cornea and produce keratitis or ulceration.

Entropion can be congenital or acquired. In addition to aging, some of the causes of acquired entropion are scarring from disorders such as trachoma, Stevens-Johnson syndrome, and mechanical, thermal, or chemical injury.

The treatment of entropion is surgery under local anesthesia. Temporary relief can be obtained by using adhesive tape to hold the skin of the lower lid down toward the cheeks, pulling the lashes off the eyeball.

Trichiasis

In trichiasis the lashes grow inward toward the eye, causing corneal irritation, erosion, and sometimes ulceration (Figure 1-2). The lid margin is not necessarily involved, as in the case of entropion. Trichiasis is often the result of scarring of the lid from injuries or severe lid inflammations.

Removing the offending cilia is temporary because they re-grow inward. Cauterization by electrolysis at the base of the lash is helpful if only a few lashes are involved. Severe cases of trichiasis require surgical removal of the entire segment of offending cilia.

Ectropion

In this condition the lid falls away from the globe (Figure 1-3). Ectropion is more common in the elderly and more often affects the lower lid. It can create corneal and conjunctival exposure with dryness and irritation. Excessive tearing, or epiphora, may result from exposure of the lacrimal punctum if the medial lid is involved.

Ectropion, either congenital or acquired, is a mechanical defect of the lids that can be remedied only by surgery. This usually involves taking a "tuck" in the lid to restore a more natural position.

Ptosis

Ptosis is a functional defect of the upper lid in which the lid margin is abnormally low because of insufficient upper eyelid retraction (Figure 1-4). This drooping of the upper lid varies in degree from hardly perceptible to complete paralysis of elevation.

Ptosis is caused by the absence or weakness of the levator palpabrae superioris muscle, and may be associated with weakness or absence of the superior rectus muscle.

Congenital ptosis is unilateral 75% of the time and is usually associated with other abnormalities such as Marcus Gunn "jaw-winking" syndrome and palsies. Acquired ptosis is common after cataract surgery in the elderly and is also associated with muscular and neurological disorders.

Treatment for ptosis is surgical. The levator palpabrae superioris muscle, the primary elevator of the lid, is shortened. Resection of this muscle and advancement of its insertion increases its leverage, pulling the lid upward.

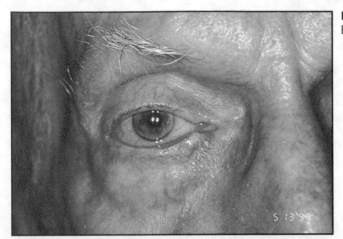

Figure 1-1. Entropion (Photograph by Angie Kasal, COT, OP).

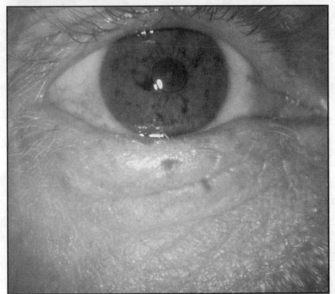

Figure 1-2. Trichiasis (Photograph by John Carswell).

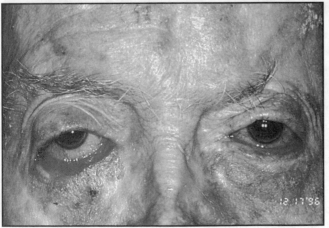

Figure 1-3. Ectropion (Photograph by Angie Kasal, COT, OP).

Figure 1-4. Ptosis (Photograph by John Carswell).

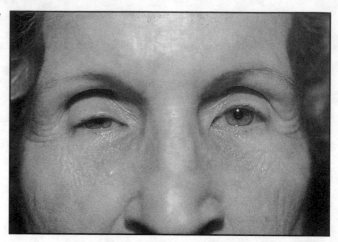

Dermatochalasis

Dermatochalasis is redundancy of eyelid skin caused by atrophy of the elastic tissue and accompanied by herniation of fat. This fold of tissue from the upper eyelid may actually hang over the lid margin, interfering with peripheral vision and causing either a true or apparent ptosis. Dermatochalasis usually occurs among older or middle-aged people, and a familial predisposition is common. Treatment is a surgical blepharoplasty with optional fat excision.

Growths

It is important to have any suspicious growths of the skin and eyelids checked by a physician. Often a biopsy is performed to determine whether or not the lesion is cancerous. Tissue is removed, fixed in a 40% formaldehyde solution, and sent to a laboratory for diagnosis.

Basal Cell Carcinoma

Basal cell carcinoma is the most common malignant tumor of the eyelids (Figure 1-5). Most of these lesions have a raised, ulcerated, pearly surface and occur on the lower lid on the inner canthus. Some have a flat and leathery appearance. This latter type is more likely to invade deeper tissues.

Treatment usually is surgical excision, although cryotherapy and radiation are sometimes used. Regrowths and metastatic spread after radiation are rare, but should be treated surgically.

Squamous Cell Carcinoma

Squamous cell carcinoma around the eyelids is much less common than basal cell, but has greater malignant potential. Squamous cell carcinoma is most common among older patients and usually develops from actinic keratoses (described on pg 5):

Treatment consists of a wide surgical excision in an attempt to remove any extensions of the growth. The lab report must include a confirmation that all margins are clear of disease.

Benign Growths

A hemangioma is a tumor composed of small dilated blood vessels. It appears as bright red dots on or near the eyelids. This congenital abnormality usually regresses with age, thus surgical removal in children is often postponed.

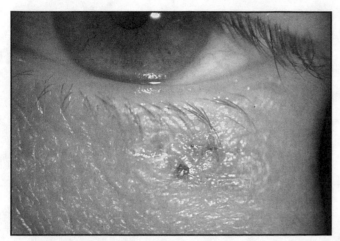

Figure 1-5. Basal cell carcinoma (Photograph by John Carswell).

Milia, or skin tags, are small, round, white, slightly elevated cysts of superficial skin appearing on the eyelids. When several milia appear together they can be perceived as a cosmetic blemish.

Nevi are flat, pigmented lesions sometimes found in eyelid tissue. They are benign and do not interfere with tissue function.

Xanthoma, or xanthelasma, are yellowish fatty deposits on the medial side of the upper and lower eyelids (Figure 1-6). They are common in the elderly and patients with high blood fat levels. Xanthoma may be eliminated by trichloracetic acid or surgery, but removal is strictly for cosmetic purposes.

Actinic keratoses, also called climatic keratopathy, are benign tumors caused by years of outdoor exposure. These precancerous lesions are usually patchy, scaly, and irregular in shape. They may be tan, ivory, or yellow in color. They should be checked regularly and removed if suspicious. Prevention is avoidance of outdoor exposure.

Infections/Inflammations

Blepharitis

OphA

Blepharitis is the most common inflammation of the eyelids and is often associated with conjunctivitis and dry eye syndrome. The lid margins become swollen, congested, and red (Figure 1-7). There is crusting around the lashes and the patient may complain of itching.

Blepharitis can be divided into two categories: anterior blepharitis, which is associated with the lashes, and posterior blepharitis, associated with the meibomian glands. Anterior blepharitis can be further classified into seborrheic or infectious inflammation. Proper and diligent lid hygiene can relieve all types of blepharitis.

Scrubbing the lids along the lash line with a good lid-scrub cleaner (or diluted no-tears baby shampoo) using a cotton-tipped applicator or warm wash cloth is helpful. After scrubbing, the cleaner should be removed by splashing water liberally on the lids.

If the etiology of blepharitis is infectious, the patient is usually given appropriate antibiotic ointment for the lids. This should be applied just before bedtime because the ointment tends to blur vision.

Figure 1-6. Xanthoma (Photograph by Angie Kasal, COT, OP).

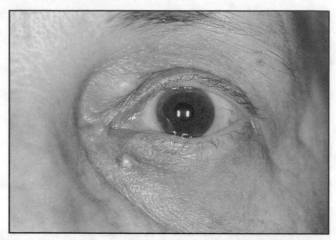

Figure 1-7. Blepharitis (Photograph by Patrick Caroline, FCLSA).

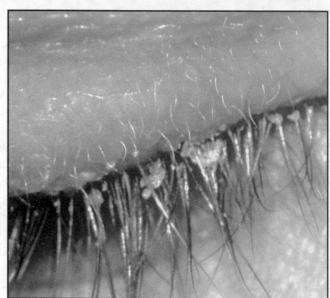

Figure 1-8. Chalazion (Photograph by Angie Kasal, COT, OP).

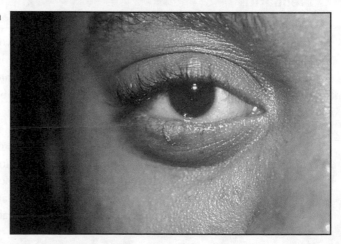

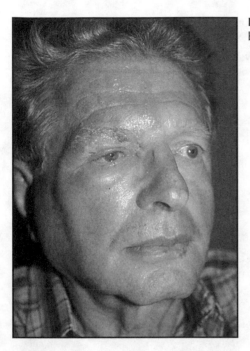

Figure 1-9. Herpes zoster ophthalmicus (Photograph by John Carswell).

Chalazion

This common disorder is a chronic inflammation of a meibomian gland located in the upper and lower lids in the area of the tarsal plates (Figure 1-8). The orifice of the meibomian gland becomes occluded, causing the lid to become swollen, painful, and inflamed before a cyst forms. Chalazia tend to be multiple and often affect the same individual again within a short period of time.

In the early stages, treatment with warm compresses is effective in most cases. If the cyst fails to resolve with compresses, it may be opened surgically and removed with a curette. Antibiotics are helpful in controlling secondary infection in the conjunctiva, but do not help the inflammation of the lid itself.

Hordeolum (Stye)

A hordeolum is an acute pustular infection of one of the small oil glands of Zeiss and Moll located in the eyelash follicles at the eyelid margins. In the early stages of infection, these glands become swollen and uncomfortable, and the lid swells. Then an abscess forms with a small collection of pus at the apex of the gland. Inflammation is usually due to invasion by the bacterium *Staphylococcus aureus*. Styes affect patients of all ages, although they are more common in young adults.

Treatment with warm compresses is effective in most cases, with topical antibiotics used to prevent secondary infections. Occasionally surgical intervention is necessary.

Herpes Zoster Ophthalmicus

This virus, also known as the chickenpox virus, affects the ophthalmic branch of the trigeminal cranial nerve. The skin area which is supplied by the affected nerve becomes extremely painful. Blister-like lesions appear on the face and sometimes involve the cornea, sclera, ciliary body, or optic nerve (Figure 1-9).

There is no satisfactory treatment, although systemically delivered cortisone and newer antiviral medications may be helpful.

Chapter 2

Lacrimal Apparatus and Orbit

- Dacryocystitis, an infection of the lacrimal sac, usually results from obstruction of the nasolacrimal duct.

- Symptoms of dacryocystitis include localized pain, edema, epiphora, and redness at the inner canthus of the eye.

- Canaliculitis is an inflammation of the lacrimal canaliculi (channels from the punctum to the nasolacrimal sac) often caused by fungal infections or secondary to dacryocystitis.

Abnormalities/Disorders/Anomalies/Growths

Lacrimal Obstruction

Nasolacrimal duct obstruction is the most common congenital abnormality of the lacrimal system. It is estimated that up to 30% of newborn infants have closure of the duct at birth. In most cases, the obstruction is resolved within 3 weeks. However, if the obstruction is not resolved, dacryocystitis (infection of the lacrimal sac) may occur. Because tears and mucus accumulate in the lacrimal sac, the sac becomes distended (Figure 2-1). Because the fluid is stagnant, bacterial infection can set up, complicating the picture.

Treatment of a lacrimal duct obstruction consists of external sac massage and application of topical antibiotics. If the obstruction is not resolved within a few weeks, the duct is probed and irrigated.

Prolapsed Tear Gland

As tissues relax with age, the lacrimal gland may drop down from its position behind the brow bone into the space between the sclera and bulbar conjunctiva (under the upper lid). The gland looks like a yellow glob which the patient sees if the upper lid is lifted. There is no pain or dysfunction of the gland. Reassurance is all that is necessary.

Exophthalmus

Exophthalmus, or proptosis, is the abnormal protrusion or bulging forward of the eyeball. Lid retraction causes the sclera to be visible between the lid margin and the limbus (scleral show). Exophthalmus may be caused from abnormalities of the thyroid gland. Occasionally, ptosis in one eye may make the other eye appear to bulge. Bilateral exophthalmus is usually due to thyroid.

Patients with exophthalmus often are unable to close the eyes completely, resulting in dry eye syndrome due to corneal exposure. Recurrent corneal erosion is often associated with incomplete closure as well.

The degree of proptosis may be recorded with an instrument called an exophthalmometer. A baseline measurement is taken and recorded for comparison with subsequent visits. (See the upcoming Basic Bookshelf Series title, *Special Skills and Techniques* for details on exophthalmometry.)

Infections/Inflammations

Dacryocystitis

Dacryocystitis is an infection of the lacrimal sac usually resulting from obstruction of the nasolacrimal duct. It occurs mostly in babies and females in their 50s. Symptoms include localized pain, edema, epiphora, and redness at the inner canthus of the eye. Applying pressure to the inner canthus may cause a reflex of purulent material.

Treatment consists of hot compresses, antibiotic drops, and systemic antibiotics. In some cases the sac is incised and drained.

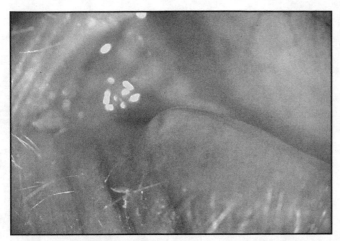

Figure 2-1. Lacrimal obstruction (Photograph by Angie Kasal, COT, OP).

Sympathetic Ophthalmia

This rare inflammation of the choroid, ciliary body, and iris is a late complication of a penetrating injury. Not only does the injured eye develop uveitis, but a similar uveitis also occurs in the other eye.

Sympathetic ophthalmia takes at least 2 weeks to appear, but is most commonly seen 2 months after the original injury. It may even take 6 months to a year before symptoms occur. Early symptoms may include slight pain, photophobia, lacrimation, disturbances in accommodation, and decreased vision.

This condition can lead to loss of vision and even blindness despite treatment with steroids. For this reason, many surgeons will enucleate a blind, injured eye within 2 weeks of the injury to avoid this dreaded complication.

Endophthalmitis

Endophthalmitis is a devastating inflammation of the intraocular tissue which occurs as a response to infection, trauma, immune reaction, or physical or chemical change. Systemic fungal infection can also cause the ocular response.

Signs and symptoms include unilateral edema, poor vision, redness of the lids and conjunctiva, and vitreous haze. The earliest sign might be an unexpected regression during the recovery period following trauma or surgery.

Aggressive treatment with an anti-fungal agent and/or antibiotic therapy is required.

Canaliculitis

Canaliculitis is an inflammation of the lacrimal canaliculi, which are tiny channels that carry tears from the conjunctiva to the tear sac. These inflammations are often caused by fungal infections or occur secondary to dacryocystitis.

Signs and symptoms may include persistent discharge, red eye, itching, epiphora, swelling and inflammation of the medial lower lid, and a "pouting" punctum. Canaliculitis may be related to allergic, bacterial, or viral infections.

Conjunctiva and Sclera

- In children, the sclera is thinner and appears bluish because of the underlying pigmented structures. In old age, the sclera may appear yellow because of the deposition of fat.

- Conjunctivitis, or "pink eye," is an inflammation of the conjunctiva. Conjunctivitis may be allergic, viral, or bacterial.

- Giant papillary conjunctivitis (GPC) is an inflammatory condition of the conjunctiva of the upper lid. GPC may be caused by soft or rigid contact lenses, postoperative stitches, prostheses, or the use of preservative-containing contact lens solutions.

Abnormalities/Disorders/Anomalies/Growths

Pinguecula

A pingueculum is a thickening of conjunctival tissue, usually just nasal to the cornea, but can also appear on the lateral side (Figure 3-1). The tissue undergoes degenerative changes and appears as a yellowish mass. Exposure to wind and dust frequently causes them, and they are often seen in older people. They usually cause no symptoms and require no treatment unless they become inflamed. (Unlike a pterygium, pinguecula never invade the cornea and are separated from the cornea by normal tissue.)

Pterygium

A pterygium is a triangular, wedge-shaped thickening of the conjunctiva beginning at the nasal or temporal border of the cornea and progressing toward the center (Figure 3-2). The tissue contains a continuation of the conjunctival epithelium and causes scarring as it invades the cornea. Pterygia that progress into the visual axis are a threat to vision.

Pterygia are degenerative in nature and are extremely common in tropical climates where people are exposed to sun, wind, and dust. Treatment for a pterygium is surgical removal, although recurrences are common.

Nevus

A nevus is a flat, pigmented, benign lesion that may be found on skin and eye tissues, including the conjunctiva (Figure 3-3). Conjunctival nevi usually appear at birth or in early childhood and become pigmented later in adolescence. It is uncommon for a conjunctival nevus to become malignant. However, an acquired pigmented lesion that occurs later (about age 40 to 50) can turn into a malignant melanoma. All conjunctival nevi should be evaluated regularly.

Scleral Degeneration

The "white of the eye" is the visible front portion of the sclera. The sclera is opaque and forms the protective outer coat of the eye. In children, the sclera is thinner and appears bluish because of the underlying pigmented structures. In old age, the sclera may appear yellow because of fat deposits. In scleral degeneration (also called hyaline degeneration), small, round, gray areas appear on the sclera anterior to the insertion of the rectus muscles (Figure 3-4). These lesions are usually 2-3 mm in diameter and cause no symptoms or complications.

Subconjunctival Hemorrhage

A subconjunctival hemorrhage (SCH) is bleeding due to a ruptured conjunctival blood vessel. It causes a bright red, but harmless, pooling of blood under the conjunctiva (Figure 3-5). It is often alarming because it appears so bright next to the white of the sclera. While it may spread at first, the blood usually absorbs within a week or 2 and no treatment is required.

Subconjunctival hemorrhages often occur in the elderly who are taking blood thinners, or are diabetic or hypertensive, but frequently no cause can be found. Sometimes they can be caused by coughing, straining, lifting, sneezing, or vomiting.

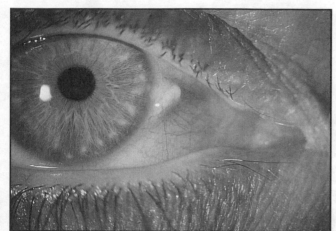

Figure 3-1. Pingueculum (Photograph by Val Sanders, COT, CRA) (Reprinted from Ledford JK, Sanders VN. *The Slit Lamp Primer.* Thorofare, NJ: SLACK Incorporated; 1998).

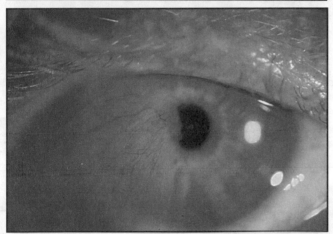

Figure 3-2. Pterygium (Photograph by Angie Kasal, COT, OP).

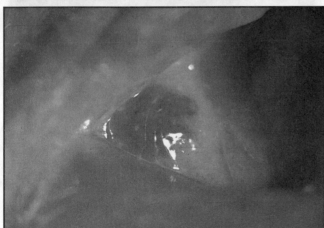

Figure 3-3. Nevus in caruncle (Photograph by John Carswell).

Figure 3-4. Scleral degeneration (Photograph courtesy of Todd Hostetter, COMT, CRA, FCLSA).

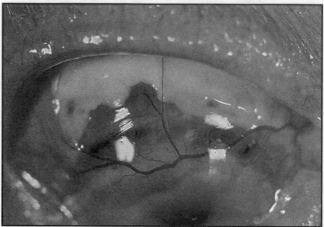

Figure 3-5. Subconjunctival hemorrhage (Photograph courtesy of Todd Hostetter, COMT, CRA, FCLSA).

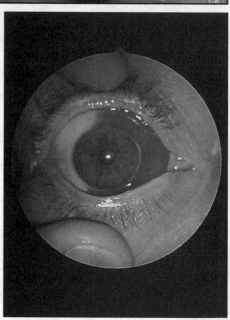

Infections/Inflammations

Conjunctivitis

Conjunctivitis, or "pink eye," is an inflammation of the conjunctiva, the mucous membrane overlying the sclera. Conjunctivitis is characterized by redness, usually greater in the fornix. Swelling occurs and there is usually a discharge that may be watery or purulent. The cornea remains clear and the pupil size is normal. There are no changes in intraocular pressure and usually no noticeable pain or photophobia. With the exception of allergic conjunctivitis, this disorder is contagious.

Allergic Conjunctivitis

Allergic conjunctivitis is basically a hypersensitivity reaction to foreign substances, sometimes associated with hay fever. It can also represent an allergy to cosmetics or a drug intolerance.

Signs and symptoms include itching, mild to moderate injection, swelling of the conjunctiva, lacrimation, and mucus discharge. Papules occur most commonly on the tarsal conjunctiva. Sodium cromoglycate and corticosteroid drops can relieve symptoms in most cases.

Vernal conjunctivitis (or vernal catarrh) is a bilateral allergic inflammation that is recurrent during warm months (Figure 3-6). The palpebral form is distinguished by cobblestone papillae on the tarsal conjunctiva. The limbal form occurs with papillary enlargement on the limbal conjunctiva associated with concretions near the limbus. The patient experiences itching, redness, lacrimation, and mucus discharge. Sodium cromoglycate and corticosteroid drops are recommended.

Viral Conjunctivitis

Several types of viral disease can cause conjunctivitis. A typical reaction includes follicles, watery discharge, and superficial punctate keratitis. Antiviral therapy is sometimes helpful, and antibiotic drops are often used to prevent secondary infection.

Adenoviruses are the most common infections of the conjunctiva. They frequently cause upper respiratory tract infections, as well as conjunctivitis, so a patient history of a cold or sore throat may be important.

The trachoma virus is associated with the Chlamydia group of microorganisms, which causes conjunctivitis that produces conjunctival follicles. Intracellular inclusion bodies can often be seen on slide specimens.

The Herpes simplex virus can produce an acute follicular conjunctivitis with painful swelling of the preauricular lymph nodes. This is usually unilateral. Small herpetic vesicles may form on the adjacent lids. The cornea is almost always involved as well (superficial punctate keratitis). (Herpetic keratitis is discussed in detail in Chapter 4.)

Bacterial Conjunctivitis

Bacterial conjunctivitis is an acute infection of the conjunctiva and may be caused by a variety of microorganisms. Bacterial conjunctivitis is characterized by a gritty sensation, conjunctival injection, and purulent discharge. The conjunctival discharge and scrapings will contain large numbers of polymorphonuclear cells, visible under the microscope.

Topical antibiotics are usually prescribed to prevent keratitis and conjunctival scarring. Patients should be advised about general hygiene measures to avoid infecting others (such as not swimming in public pools and not sharing face towels).

Giant Papillary Conjunctivitis (GPC)

OphA

Giant papillary conjunctivitis refers to an inflammatory condition of the conjunctiva of the upper lid in which the papillae reach a diameter of 1 mm or more (Figure 3-7). The tissue generally becomes swollen and irritated. GPC can be caused by soft or rigid contact lenses, postoperative stitches, prostheses, or the use of contact lens solutions containing preservatives.

GPC is graded in four stages. (Since GPC is most often associated with contact lens wear, we will assume that situation here.) The early symptoms include mild itching and awareness of the lenses. Advanced symptoms include extreme itching or pain, mucus accumulation, blurring, and

Figure 3-6. Vernal conjunctivitis (Photograph courtesy of Todd Hostetter, COMT, CRA, FCLSA).

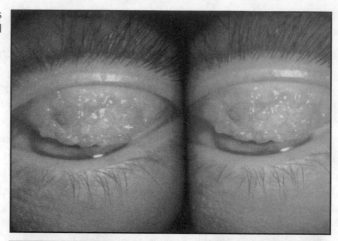

Figure 3-7. GPC (Photograph by Val Sanders, COT, CRA) (Reprinted from Ledford JK, Sanders VN. *The Slit Lamp Primer.* Thorofare, NJ: SLACK Incorporated; 1998).

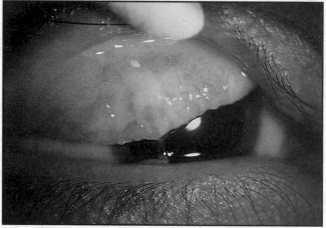

excess movement of the contact lens. Advanced signs include moderate to severe contact lens coating, red eyes, giant papillae, and corneal punctate staining. The observation of increased mucus levels is one of the most important signs in the diagnosis of GPC.

Treatment of GPC can be exasperating. Contact lens patients with GPC should have their care regimes evaluated, keeping in mind that all contact lens solutions containing preservatives can contribute to the problem. Often, changing the type of lens a patient is wearing can be helpful. A rigid gas permeable (RGP) lens is recommended. Soft lenses should include a non-HEMA choice if possible, or at least a thin, low-water type. Disposables and frequent replacement lenses are also possible options.

Episcleritis

Episcleritis is an inflammation of the fibro-elastic vascular tissue that overlies the surface of the sclera (Figure 3-8). There are two forms. Simple episcleritis, the most common, is associated with inflammatory medical conditions. It is characterized by a very acute onset, is usually mild, and resolves rapidly. Nodular episcleritis is a raised area of inflammation, usually near the limbus. The nodules may be single or multiple, and the condition is usually recurrent. Topical steroids will speed up the process of resolution in both conditions.

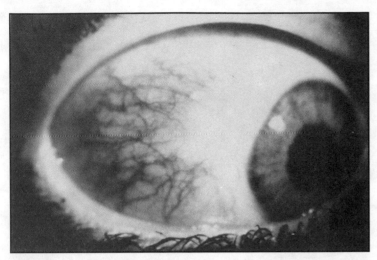

Figure 3-8. Episcleritis (note raised nodule) (Reprinted from Ledford JK, Sanders VN. *The Slit Lamp Primer.* Thorofare, NJ: SLACK Incorporated; 1998).

Scleritis

Scleritis is an inflammation of the collagen and elastic tissue of the sclera and episclera. Scleritis causes severe pain to the patient and actually destroys tissue, sometimes the entire eye. Scleral thinning and necrosis occurs in most cases. Causes or associated systemic conditions of scleritis include keratitis, uveitis, glaucoma, cataract, and retinal detachment.

Systemic nonsteroid antiinflammatory agents (NSAIDs) and topical steroids are used to treat scleritis. In severe cases systemic steroids are necessary.

Chapter 4

Cornea

KEY POINTS

- Corneal dystrophy, a process in which a mature tissue undergoes atrophy or regression, results in cloudiness of the cornea and a reduction in vision.

- Keratoconus, a degenerative disease causing the central cornea to thin and bulge forward, causes irregular astigmatism.

- Arcus senilis is a benign degenerative corneal change that causes a gray-white ring which encircles the corneal limbus.

- Corneal ulcers may be caused by bacterial, fungal, or viral infections, and chemical or physical insults.

- Corneal edema (or swelling) is caused by a disturbance in the endothelium's pump action or damage to corneal layers (especially the endothelium) causing a buildup of fluid in the tissues.

- Keratoconjunctivitis sicca (KCS) is a dry eye situation that affects much of the population.

Abnormalities/Disorders/Anomalies/Growths

Corneal Dystrophy

Corneal dystrophy is the process in which the mature corneal tissue undergoes atrophy or regression (Figure 4-1). The abnormality is inherited and usually shows up later in life. Various dystrophies affect different layers of the cornea, but all result in cloudiness of the cornea and reduced vision.

Epithelial Dystrophy

Cogan's microcystic epithelial dystrophy (also called epithelial basement membrane dystrophy or fingerprint-map-dot dystrophy) is the most common anterior membrane corneal dystrophy (Figure 4-2). Although no definitive hereditary pattern has been recognized, the disease is dominantly inherited and occurs in both sexes. Some studies indicate as much as 76% of the population over the age of 50 is affected. This dystrophy seems often to affect caucasian women.

Cogan's dystrophy is probably a result of the synthesis of abnormal basement membrane tissue. This causes a thickening of the membrane with extensions into the epithelium and fibrous material between the membrane and Bowman's layer. (Transient basement membrane lesions lasting less than 3 months are seen in about 75% of patients following radial keratotomy.)

Symptoms of severe pain on waking in the morning, photophobia, and slightly reduced visual acuity can be related to recurrent corneal erosions associated with the dystrophy. Dots, maps, and fingerprint opacities tend to come and go spontaneously. The dots are large gray cysts or fine blebs; the maps are diffuse gray lesions that contain clear oval areas and vary greatly in size. The fingerprints may stain with fluorescein. Irregular astigmatism rarely develops and visual loss is usually minimal. The recurrent erosions require treatment by double-patching the eye for 48 hours so that the defect will epithelialize, followed by a bland hypertonic ointment at night for a few weeks. Superficial epithelial keratectomy and soft bandage lenses relieve symptoms for some patients. Penetrating keratoplasty is the only treatment for very advanced cases.

Meesmann's epithelial dystrophy begins in the first decade of life as tiny, round, clear vesicles in the epithelium. There may be some surface irregularities, but between the vesicles the cornea remains clear. They may be seen by direct illumination or retroillumination. The patient usually remains asymptomatic until the fourth or fifth decade when the cysts break through to the surface, causing irregular astigmatism, pain, epiphora, and photophobia.

Bowman's Layer Dystrophy

Reis-Bücklers' dystrophy is a corneal dystrophy of Bowman's layer usually appearing in the first decade of life as a superficial corneal opacification associated with painful recurrent erosion. The erosions usually occur up to 3 or 4 times a year and cause severe pain, photophobia, and ocular hyperemia. By the fourth decade they become less frequent, corneal sensation decreases, and the corneal surface becomes irregular. This irregularity causes a great visual disability for the patient.

The recurrent erosions of Reis-Bücklers' dystrophy can be treated with hypertonic drops during the day and hypertonic ointment at night with patching, debridement, or soft contact lenses. In patients with severe disease, keratoplasty is necessary.

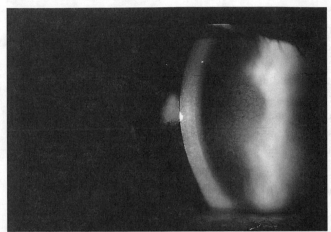

Figure 4-1. Corneal dystrophy (Photograph by Val Sanders, COT, CRA) (Reprinted from Ledford JK, Sanders VN. The Slit Lamp Primer. Thorofare, NJ: SLACK Incorporated; 1998).

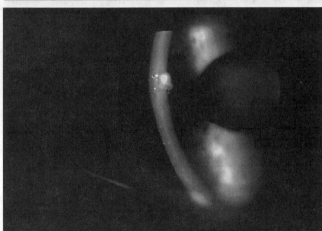

Figure 4-2. Map-dot and Fuch's dystrophy which affect the epithelial layer of the cornea (Photograph by Val Sanders, COT, CRA).

Stromal Dystrophy

Granular dystrophy causes white opacities to appear in the superficial stroma of the central cornea in the first decade of life. The stroma between the lesions remains clear until the condition progresses and the opacities enlarge and increase in number. This bilateral disease only affects the central cornea. No treatment is required in the early stages, but as the disease progresses penetrating keratoplasty may be necessary to restore vision.

Lattice dystrophy causes small refractile lines, anterior stromal white dots, subepithelial opacities, and faint central haze in the anterior stroma. These appear in the first decade of life. The lattice lines slowly develop and become larger, thicker, and more opaque. With time, the tissue between the lines becomes hazy.

Patients with lattice dystrophy have recurrent erosions, pain, photophobia, and redness. Treatments include hypertonic drops during the day and hypertonic ointment at night with patching, debridement, or soft contact lenses. In patients with severe disease, keratoplasty is necessary.

Endothelial Dystrophy

Posterior polymorphous dystrophy is a bilateral, dominantly transmitted endothelial corneal dystrophy. The lesions usually appear in clusters of two to twenty. When viewed by retro-illumination, the entire posterior cornea has an "orange peel" appearance. This is usually a nonprogressive condition. However, in some cases, symptoms of decreased visual acuity and corneal edema can be severe enough to warrant keratoplasty.

Fuch's dystrophy (or epithelial-endothelial dystrophy) is a bilateral central corneal disease. Pigment dusting and guttatae appear in the posterior cornea in the early phase of the disease. Descemet's membrane is opaque and thickened. Patients experience photophobia and hazy vision as the edema worsens. Small, clear cysts begin to appear in the epithelium, causing irregular astigmatism. Eventually, large bullae appear and rupture, causing pain.

Soft bandage contact lenses are sometimes effective, but penetrating keratoplasty is indicated when visual acuity is reduced to an unacceptable level.

Keratoconus (Ectactic Dystrophy)

Keratoconus is a degenerative disease that causes the central cornea to thin and bulge forward. Keratoconus may be congenital, but often manifests at puberty or shortly thereafter. It is usually bilateral. Ectasia (stretching) progresses at varying rates and may remain stable for long periods of time. The cone may be round, ripple'shaped, or oval, and its apex is usually located inferiorly and nasally. If the ectasia affects the entire cornea, the condition is called keratoglobus.

Early symptoms of keratoconus include decreased vision (usually manifested as an increase in myopia and astigmatism). As the disease progresses, thinning at the apex of the cornea occurs, as well as a reduction of corneal sensitivity. Ruptures in Bowman's membrane produce linear scars that may interfere with vision. Ophthalmic examination will reveal myopic astigmatism (during refractometry), Fleisher's iron ring and apical thinning (with the slit lamp), and a scissors reflex (with the retinoscope). There are also irregular and steepening keratometer mires, and irregular rings with Placido's disk. Corneal topography is helpful in diagnosing keratoconus. In advanced keratoconus, the cone will push the lower lid out when the patient looks down. This is known as Munson's sign.

Treatment for keratoconus includes wearing rigid gas permeable contact lenses to correct the irregular astigmatism. Some practitioners believe that rigid lenses will hinder progression of the cone, but this is debatable. Penetrating keratoplasty may be needed if the patient cannot tolerate the contact lens or if too much scarring has occurred. Although recurrence of keratoconus in a graft has been reported, the prognosis of penetrating keratoplasty is extremely good.

Krukenberg's Spindle

Krukenberg's spindle is vertical pigment deposits in the central portion of the endothelium. It is a clinical sign resulting from pigment dispersion glaucoma and sometimes follows uveitis. It can also be benign.

Corneal Scarring

The epithelial layer of the cornea (including its basement layer) and Descemet's membrane regenerate without scarring after injury. Bowman's membrane and the stroma do not regenerate when damaged. A permanent scar or opacity is the result of injury of these deeper tissues (Figure 4-3). In addition, trauma to the endothelium usually results in a decrease in cell density.

Trauma to the cornea can result in irregular astigmatism. This corneal irregularity cannot be corrected with glasses. (Refractive surgery is actually controlled scarring to correct the refractive error.) A rigid contact lens is required for visual rehabilitation. If scarring occurs in the visual

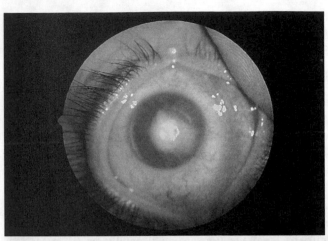

Figure 4-3. Corneal scarring (Photograph courtesy of Todd Hostetter, COMT, CRA, FCLSA).

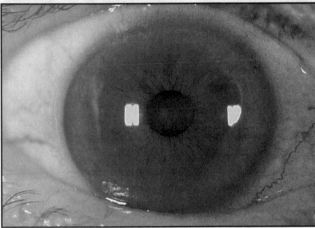

Figure 4-4. Arcus senilis (Photograph courtesy of Todd Hostetter, COMT, CRA, FCLSA).

axis, smoothing the cornea with a rigid lens may not correct the patient's vision and a corneal graft may be necessary.

Arcus Senilis

Arcus senilis, also called gerontoxan, is a degenerative corneal change that causes a gray-white ring which circles the corneal limbus (Figure 4-4). It is basically a benign deposit of fat typically seen in patients older than 60 and in young patients with high blood fat levels.

Infections/Inflammations

Keratitis

Keratitis, or inflammation of the cornea, may be caused by bacteria, virus, fungus, or exposure. The cornea will exhibit a loss of luster and transparency, and cellular infiltration will be noted. Keratitis is often accompanied by conjunctivitis and all its symptoms. Lesions are most easily recognized on slit lamp examination with the cobalt blue filter after staining with fluorescein.

Bacterial Keratitis

Bacterial keratitis usually tends to occur after injury to the epithelium or in the compromised cornea. Stromal infiltration, edema, folds, and anterior chamber reaction indicate microbial infection.

Staphylococcus is the most common bacteria seen with localized ulcers. *Pneumococcus* is less defined and associated with a hypopyon. *Pseudomonas* is a very rapid, destructive keratitis.

Acanthamoeba Keratitis

Acanthamoeba are free-living protozoa, and infections are rare; only a few hundred cases have been reported. However, acanthamoeba keratitis should be suspected in patients with a history of minor corneal trauma (Figure 4-5). Unlike bacterial infections, which generally resolve after a few days of treatment, this infection persists for months and is usually associated with severe pain.

In the early stages, diagnosis can be made relatively easily by microscopic examination of tissue that has been removed by scraping the epithelium and culturing the organism. The progress from epithelial disease to stromal disease is rapid. Therefore, early diagnosis is important, since treatment is easier when the disease is limited to the epithelium.

OptA

Acanthamoeba can be found in swimming environments and in non-sterile solutions or rinses. The infection is more common in contact lens wearers, but contact lens-related occurrences have decreased since the practice of making saline with salt tablets and distilled water has been largely discontinued. Contact lens disinfectants with low concentrations of biocides appear to be useful for retarding acanthamoeba without ocular surface toxicity.

Viral Keratitis

Viruses are often implicated in keratitis. Examples are Herpes simplex and Herpes zoster. They produce a foreign body sensation associated with epiphora and blepharospasm. Fluorescein staining of the resulting corneal ulcer usually reveals a branch-like, dendritic pattern (Figure 4-6).

Treatment involves the instillation of antibiotic ointment such as polymyxin-bacitracin or gentamicin and a short-acting cycloplegic. The eye is patched for 24-48 hours, then topical antibiotic ointment or drops 2-3 times per day should be continued for 4 days to protect against infection. Treatment may also include topical antiviral medication.

Fungal Keratitis

Corneal inflammation can also be caused by fungi. *Candida* is the most common yeast fungi. It often occurs in eyes where there has been chronic use of corticosteroids. Exposure keratitis, keratitis sicca, herpes simplex keratitis, and prior keratoplasty are also risk factors. *Candida* is common in the northern and coastal regions of the United States.

The most common filamentous fungi are *Fusarium, Cephalospovium,* and *Aspergillus*. These usually infect following mild abrasive corneal trauma, especially after injury from vegetable matter. Fungal infection of the eye poses a significant threat, not only due to the potential damage, but also because of the limited number of approved antifungal agents available for treatment.

The most important step in early diagnosis is prompt scraping and laboratory analysis. Approved antifungal drugs and cycloplegics should be used liberally. If medical treatment fails, debridement and superficial keratectomy may be indicated. Severe fungal keratitis can be so serious that it causes death.

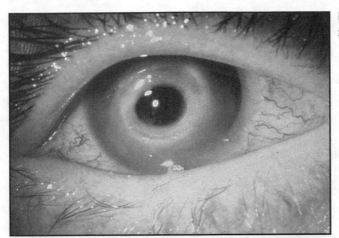

Figure 4-5. Acanthamoeba (Photograph by Patrick Caroline, FCLSA).

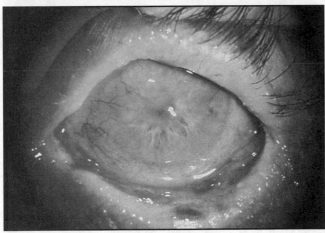

Figure 4-6. Viral (Herpes Zoster) Keratitis (Photograph by Patrick Caroline, FCLSA).

Exposure Keratitis

Exposure keratitis is the result of corneal drying due to incomplete closure of the eyelid. Corneal irritation, then inflammation, result from the loss of corneal wetting and lubrication, most often in the inferior portion of the cornea.

Exposure keratitis is often caused by neurological problems associated with a seventh (facial) nerve palsy.

Frequent instillation of artificial tears during the day and lubricating ointment at night (with taping the eyelid closed) is helpful in mild cases of exposure keratitis. Moderate exposure may require a soft bandage lens. Severe cases require aggressive therapy, including high dose systemic steroids.

Ulcers

Corneal ulcers can be caused by bacterial, fungal, or viral infections, and chemical or physical insults. Initial destruction of the epithelium and Bowman's layer is followed by destruction of the stroma, which can be massive. Ulceration with superficial white infiltrates is commonly seen in bacterial ulcers. Dendritic, branch-like lesions are seen with viral ulcers.

Figure 4-7. Bacterial (*Pseudomonas*) ulcer (Photograph by Phyllis Rakow, FCLSA, COMT).

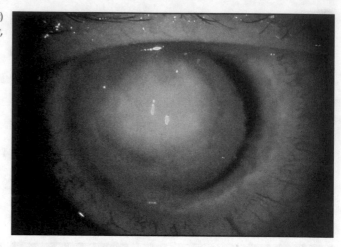

OptT

Bacterial Ulcers

Bacterial infections are a common and potentially dangerous form of corneal ulceration (Figure 4-7). *Pseudomonas aeruginosa, Staphylococcus aureus, pneumococcus, streptococcus* and *Escherichia coli* are often the culprits. Bacterial ulcers are common following eye injuries when there has been a break in the epithelium, especially if the cornea was exposed to organic material.

Usually, specific diagnosis requires identifying the organism by culture or by gram staining of tissue sections. Cultures are used to determine the appropriate antibiotic, but usually a broad spectrum antibiotic is used while waiting for culture results.

Pseudomonas aeruginosa is a most dangerous organism. It thrives in moist places, needing only a trace of organic material to survive, and has been known to prefer fluorescein. Because of this, fluorescein-impregnated paper strips have replaced most fluorescein solutions. The organism cannot survive in a dry environment. Medical practices should be particular to avoid contamination of all ophthalmic solutions, including antibiotics.

Fungal Ulcers

Corneal ulceration caused by fungi usually occurs after trauma involving vegetable material. An unexplained delay in healing of a corneal ulcer may indicate the presence of a fungal keratitis (Figure 4-8). After an injury, the onset of the ulcer is usually seen in 8 to 15 days. Common fungal organisms are *Candida albicans, Aspergillus, Cephalosporium, Fusarium*, and *Mucorales*. Appearance is similar to the bacterial ulcer and a hypopyon is almost always present.

Viral Ulcers

The most frequent type of virus-induced corneal ulcer results from the Herpes simplex type I virus. These ulcers are branched-shaped lesions called dendrites, which affect the corneal epithelium with or without involvement of the stroma (Figure 4-9). Dendritic ulcers usually affect the central cornea and, therefore, have great potential for visual damage. They tend to recur once the virus is in the body.

Herpes zoster dendritic ulcers are less common. They may occur after a cold, an infectious disease (typhoid fever, malaria), fever therapy, vaccination, menstruation, or trauma. The lesions are usually painful. The healing process may take weeks or months. Verification of the diagnosis can be confirmed by corneal scrapings and Giemsa staining, or by laboratory examination of excised tissue.

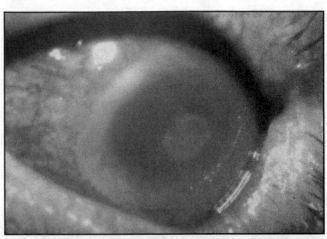

Figure 4-8. Fungal ulcer (Photograph by Patrick Caroline, FCLSA).

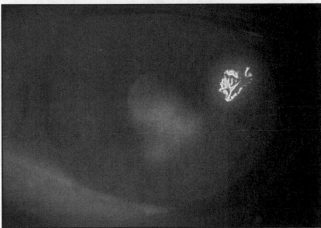

Figure 4-9. Dendritic (viral) ulcer (Photograph by John Carswell).

Corneal Edema

Corneal edema is swelling of the cornea (Figure 4-10). The normal cornea remains clear because of the action of the endothelial layer. A disturbance in the endothelium's pump action or damage to corneal layers (especially the endothelium) causes a buildup of fluid in the tissues, causing swelling.

Mild cases of epithelial edema cause a decrease in transparency of the epithelium, appearing as a diffuse haze. Moderate cases appear as fine intraepithelial vesicles, and as bullae in severe cases (Figure 4-11). Normal eye and lid movements may result in painful rupture of the bullae. Patients experience photophobia, halos around lights, redness, and discomfort.

Edema of Bowman's layer usually accompanies edematous changes in the epithelium and stroma. Stromal edema occurs in conjunction with corneal trauma, inflammation, degeneration, metabolic abnormalities, and glaucoma. The stroma's thickness increases as a result of the accumulation of fluid and, often, to the influx of acute inflammatory cells as well. The stroma appears hazy when viewed with the slit lamp. This stromal haze is related to diffraction of light induced by irregularities in the stroma's lamellar alignment.

Descemet's membrane is normally inconspicuous; only in its diseased state are irregularities apparent. Because of its proximity to the stroma and the endothelium, Descemet's membrane reflects stromal edema by developing irregular folds.

The endothelium normally loses cells with age and the remaining cells tend to thin out and

Figure 4-10. Corneal edema (Photograph by Val Sanders, COT, CRA) (Reprinted from Ledford JK, Sanders VN. *The Slit Lamp Primer.* Thorofare, NJ: SLACK Incorporated; 1998).

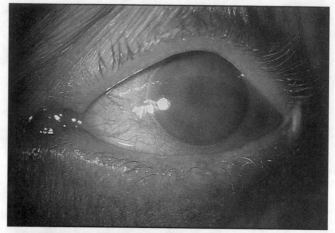

Figure 4-11. Microcystic edema (Photograph by Patrick Caroline, FCLSA).

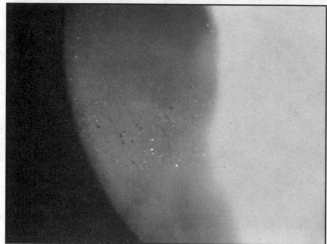

spread. This degeneration contributes to corneal edema. Other causes of endothelial edema are Fuch's and other dystrophies, surgical and nonsurgical trauma, glaucoma, keratitis, and uveitis.

Keratoconjunctivitis Sicca (KCS)

OphA

OptA

In dry eye, also known as keratoconjunctivitis sicca (KCS), the cornea's smooth surface is altered because there are not enough tears or wetting ability to create or support a smooth refractive surface (Figure 4-12). Symptoms may include a sandy-gritty irritation, redness, photophobia, mucus strands, foreign body sensation, and contact lens intolerance.

Superficial punctate staining of the cornea and conjunctiva is seen in patients with KCS. There is often an increased frequency of chalazia, blepharitis, 3 & 9 o'clock staining, mucus strands in the lower cul-de-sac, and filaments on the cornea. When these filaments (which are strands of coiled, superficial corneal epithelium) break loose, they leave behind small, painful corneal ulcers.

Tear production normally decreases with age (60% lower at age 65 than at age 18). Dry eye occurs in males and females, but is seen most often in post-menopausal females because of the lack of estrogen. Suspect dry eye in patients over 40 if there is presence of rose bengal staining, a diminished tear meniscus, and a Schirmer strip test result less than 5 mm.

Systemic medications often contribute to KCS. Known to cause such problems are diuretics,

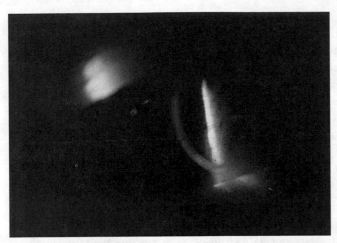

Figure 4-12. Keratoconjunctivitis Sicca (KCS) stained with rose bengal (Photograph by Val Sanders, COT, CRA) (Reprinted from Ledford JK, Sanders VN. *The Slit Lamp Primer*. Thorofare, NJ: SLACK Incorporated; 1998).

belladonna tranquilizers, antihistimines, birth control pills, blood pressure medications, and acne medications. Any medication whose purpose is to decrease body fluids (whether sinus secretions or water) will generally dry the tear film as well.

Systemic diseases associated with dry eye include Sjogren's syndrome, rheumatoid arthritis, lupus, and thyroid imbalance. Corneal exposure should be suspected as a cause for dry eye symptoms in patients with lid abnormalities or nerve/muscle problems that prevent the lids from closing completely. Taping the lid closed may be helpful in these cases.

Contact lenses exacerbate KCS. Contact lenses ride on the tear film layer, and a compromised tear film makes lens wear less comfortable and can cause further corneal damage. Lower water content soft lenses tend to be more comfortable, and gas permeable lenses are usually recommended over soft lenses for dry eye patients. These patients tend to tolerate the lens better with shorter wearing times and liberal use of tear supplements, preferably non-preserved.

There are four primary methods of diagnosing KCS. They are the tear break-up time (BUT), Schirmer test, rose bengal staining method, and phenol red thread test.

BUT stands for tear (film) break-up time. Between blinks, the tears evaporate as the tear film thins. Dry spots develop, exposing the corneal epithelium. Blinking again restores the tear film and covers the dry spot. The BUT is an evaluation of tear film stability by measuring the interval of time between the last complete blink and the development of the first dry spot. Fluorescein dye and the cobalt blue filter are used to facilitate this observation. Normal tear BUT is 15 to 45 seconds; a dry eye or a mucin-deficient dry eye will break up in 5 to 10 seconds. Look for pathology at sites that tend to dry with every blink. In addition, the shorter the break-up time, the more likely the patient will have problems with soft contact lenses.

The Schirmer test is the standard measurement for aqueous tear production. Strips of filter paper are placed in the patient's lower cul-de-sac and the amount of the moisture on the strip is measured after 5 minutes. The test can be performed with or without anesthesia. Less than 3 mm of moistening with anesthesia and less than 4 mm without anesthesia is highly indicative of decreased aqueous tear production. When the results are more than 15 mm, the aqueous tear production could be normal or could represent reflex tearing, giving a false impression.

Rose bengal stains devitalized epithelial cells red, aiding in the diagnosis of KCS. Mucus and filaments on the surface of the cornea and conjunctiva will stain as well.

The new standard measurement for testing aqueous tear production is the phenol red thread test. It is similar to the Schirmer test. A red cotton thread is placed in the patient's lower cul-de-sac, and the amount of wetting (represented by a color change) is measured in 15 seconds. This test seems to induce less reflex tearing, and requires less time to perform.

The liberal use of tear supplements (preservative free is preferred) and night time ointment may be helpful in rehabilitating a compromised tear film. Vitamin therapy is an interesting and controversial attempt to improve symptoms of KCS. Some practicioners feel that Vitamin A supplements are helpful.

Humidifiers often relieve dry eye symptoms, as well as avoidance of moving air (fans, etc) and smoke. Goggle-type glasses may be used in an effort to eliminate evaporation by creating moisture traps in front of the eye; their drawback is the lack of social acceptance.

Lacriserts (Merck & Co, Inc, West Point, Pa) are rod-shaped, water-soluble pellets made of hydroxypropyl cellulose (5 mg). One is inserted into the inferior cul-de-sac of the eye daily to relieve the symptoms associated with moderate to severe dry eye syndromes.

Punctual occlusion is sometimes used to increase the lacrimal lake and help keep tears from draining through the punctum. Temporary punctal occlusion with silicone plugs is suggested before permanent occlusion to verify a successful reduction in dry eye symptoms. Permanent occlusion can be performed by electrocautery or laser.

Neovascularization

Neovascularization is the growth of blood vessels from the limbal area into the cornea (Figure 4-13). There are two types of corneal vascularization—superficial and deep. Superficial vascularization occurs by ingrowth of a pannus from the limbus. (See next section.) Deep vascularization is a common result of keratitis. Severe cases of neovascularization, where vessel encroachment extends further into the cornea, are rare and seen most often superiorly, under the upper lid. If the vessels extend into the optical zone, scarring can occur.

Neovascularization can be caused by varying degrees of hypoxia, and is often associated with soft contact lens wear.

OptA

Patients with corneal disease such as Fuch's dystrophy or keratoconus must be watched closely after penetrating keratoplasty, because vascularization can threaten the donor cornea.

Resolved vascularization leaves vessel walls (ghost vessels), which never regress. Although no new vessels may be formed, the old vessels may become easily engorged with blood. Initial evaluation of patients should include careful evaluation for vessels from previous episodes of neovascularization.

Pannus

Pannus is abnormal blood vessels and fibrous tissue that infiltrate the cornea (Figure 4-14). Degenerative pannus is associated with late chronic bullous keratopathy, and inflammatory pannus with trachoma. The vascular connective tissue of the pannus arises from the conjunctiva. Pannus often destroys Bowman's layer, but usually the degenerative changes tend to remain in the epithelium.

Guttata

Guttata are small "wart-like" deposits on Descemet's membrane that are abnormal products of the endothelial cells (Figure 4-15). Guttata are usually seen in patients over 40 years of age. They can compromise or destroy endothelial cells, causing a compromise in the metabolic

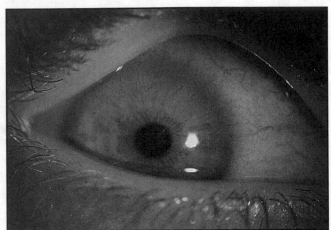

Figure 4-13. Corneal vascularization (Photograph by Val Sanders, COT, CRA) (Reprinted from Ledford JK, Sanders VN. *The Slit Lamp Primer.* Thorofare, NJ: SLACK Incorporated; 1998).

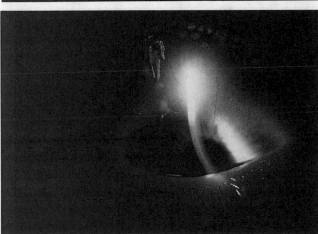

Figure 4-14. Corneal pannus (Photograph by Val Sanders, COT, CRA) (Reprinted from Ledford JK, Sanders VN. *The Slit Lamp Primer.* Thorofare, NJ: SLACK Incorporated; 1998).

process and stromal edema, followed by epithelial edema and bullous keratopathy. The average case of guttata remains moderate and stationary for years. Severe types of guttata are associated with Fuch's dystrophy.

Infiltrates

An infiltrate is a subepithelial accumulation of inflammatory cells and extracellular material within the corneal tissue, usually just below the epithelial layer (Figure 4-16). They can also be located in the stroma. Infiltrates are usually grayish-white, and signs of infection are mild and localized. They may appear punctuate, oval, or stellate (like a starburst). Under the slit lamp, the area of insult can range from semi-opaque to opaque under direct illumination and is also visible with retroillumination.

Infiltrates usually do not stain. Unlike an ulcer in which the epithelium is attacked from the outside (creating a depression), an infiltrate creates a slightly raised lesion due to the internal accumulation of inflammatory cells. An epithelial break that will take up fluorescein stain may occur if the lesion implodes. Infectious infiltrates often develop as a result of infectious keratitis.

Corneal infiltrates may be sterile (ie, not caused by microorganisms) or infectious. Infected infiltrates can be caused by any infective keratitis. Sterile infiltrates can be caused by allergies, viruses, or chemical toxicity from contact lens solutions.

Figure 4-15. Corneal guttatae (Photograph courtesy of Val Sanders, COT, CRA).

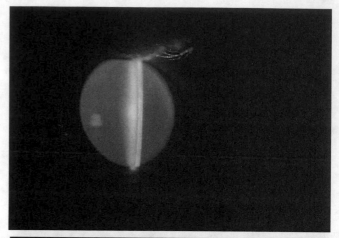

Figure 4-16. Subepithelial infiltrates (seen in epidemic keratoconjunctivitis) (Photograph by Val Sanders, COT, CRA) (Reprinted from Ledford JK, Sanders VN. *The Slit Lamp Primer.* Thorofare, NJ: SLACK Incorporated; 1998).

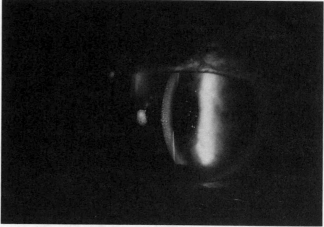

Infectious infiltrates tend to be associated with pain, photophobia, discharge, hyperemia, and anterior chamber reactions. On the other hand, sterile infiltrates are associated with minimal discomfort, little anterior chamber reaction, absence of corneal staining, and no discharge.

Chapter 5

Glaucoma Overview

KEY POINTS

- Glaucoma is the condition in which the pressure in the eye is elevated enough to result in optic nerve damage and visual field loss. All three of these elements are required for the diagnosis of glaucoma.

- Glaucoma is the third leading cause of blindness in the United States.

- Although approximately 15 million Americans have glaucoma, about one million are unaware of it.

- Risk factors for glaucoma include high intraocular pressure (IOP), advanced age, being of African descent, family history of glaucoma, myopia, diabetes, and high blood pressure.

- The goal in treatment of the patient with glaucoma is to control intraocular pressure and strive to eliminate, or at least minimize, damage to the patient's vision.

Aqueous and Intraocular Pressure

The anterior chamber of the eye (between the cornea and iris) and the posterior chamber of the eye (between the back of the iris and including the lens) are both filled with a watery fluid known as the aqueous humor (or aqueous). The aqueous is similar in composition to blood plasma, and is formed by the ciliary body at the root of the iris. From here, it circulates in front of the lens and through the pupil, into the anterior chamber. The aqueous then drains out of the eye at the angle, which is the place where the cornea meets the iris. The angle is made up of a net-like structure called the trabecular meshwork (or trabeculum). From the trabeculum, the aqueous flows into the canal of Schlemm and then into capillaries. The capillaries release the aqueous into the bloodstream.

Because the aqueous is constantly being formed and drained out, there is an equilibrium of pressure (known as intraocular pressure, or IOP) inside the eye. If too much aqueous is formed or the aqueous does not drain out properly, then the IOP will rise. If the IOP rises high enough and stays elevated for a significant period of time, the pressure can cause irreparable damage to the optic nerve (and thus, to the patient's vision).

IOP is measured with a tonometer, which gives a pressure reading in millimeters of mercury (mm Hg). Just what qualifies as "normal" IOP is debated among experts. Generally speaking, normal pressure is between 13 and 19 mm Hg, but this reading can vary significantly among individuals. The pressure can even vary in the same person throughout the day, with the highest readings usually occurring in early morning (around 7 am) and lowest readings in the evening. The difference between the am and pm readings may vary from 5 to 15 mm Hg.

When the amount of aqueous exceeds the draining ability of the eye (for whatever reason), the IOP is elevated. This puts undue pressure on the tissues of the eye. The structure that is most affected is the optic nerve. If the elevated pressure is sustained for long enough periods, the nerve fibers of the optic nerve may be damaged or even destroyed. This, in turn, causes a change in the patient's peripheral vision. When the triad of elevated IOP, nerve damage, and peripheral vision loss occur together, the condition is diagnosed as glaucoma. In almost every case of glaucoma, outflow abnormality from the anterior chamber (rather than above-normal rates of aqueous humor production) is the reason for increased IOP.

Types of Glaucoma

Glaucoma may be classified as open-angle, with primary and secondary types, or angle-closure, also with primary and secondary types.

In open-angle glaucoma, the aqueous humor has full access to the angle of the anterior chamber, but there is abnormally high resistance to the fluid flow through the trabecular meshwork and Schlemm's canal. There is no interference of the peripheral iris to the draining angle structures.

Primary open-angle glaucoma, the most common form of glaucoma, is a silent non-symptomatic disease, not secondary to another disease or condition. Gradual loss of peripheral vision occurs first, and central vision is affected only in the late stages. Only by measuring IOP and examining the optic nerve head with the ophthalmoscope can open-angle glaucoma be detected in its early stages.

Secondary open-angle glaucoma occurs as a result of another eye disease or condition (such as uveitis or trauma), resulting in secondary blockage or damage to the canals or collector channels.

In angle-closure glaucoma, the aqueous humor is prevented access to the trabecular meshwork because of a peripheral iris blockage. Angle-closure glaucoma can be intermittent. Acute symptoms can be reversed when the peripheral iris is moved away from the angle's draining structures. In angle-closure glaucoma, the trabecular meshwork and Schlemm's canal usually have normal resistance to fluid flow. The IOP is only elevated when the peripheral iris covers the trabecular meshwork. Symptoms include pain (may be severe), redness, burred vision, and halos around lights.

In primary angle-closure glaucoma, relative pupillary block is the mechanism of angle closure. There is resistance to the aqueous humor flow between the posterior iris surface and lens due to their close proximity at the pupil. Shallowness of the anterior chamber can be an indication of the potential for possible angle-closure glaucoma.

Secondary angle-closure glaucoma is related to another eye disease or condition (such as a swollen cataract or diabetic neovascularization) that prevents aqueous flow throughout the chamber.

Evaluation for Glaucoma

An examination for glaucoma involves evaluation of the depth of the anterior chamber using a flashlight or slit lamp. The slit lamp exam should also include scanning for the presence of inflammatory cells (keratitic precipitates) on the corneal epithelium, anterior chamber cells and flare, iris vessels, and lens surface exfoliation. Intraocular pressure should be taken with applanation or Schiotz tonometry. An IOP of more than 22 should be considered suspicious. Optic atrophy of the disk (disk cupping) should be noted. A visual field test should be performed, and the angle should be evaluated with gonioscopy. Glaucoma suspects should be seen frequently to evaluate disease progression.

Because of the pattern of optic nerve fiber destruction, glaucoma typically produces a nerve fiber bundle defect (an arcuate defect or Bjerrum scotoma) or a nasal step defect in the visual field. This change usually goes unnoticed by the patient. Central changes occur later as the disease progresses.

LV

Treatment

Medications (usually topical and sometimes oral) are used to control IOP. Pilocarpine and carbachol are used in chronic open-angle glaucoma to increase the facility of aqueous outflow. Epinephrine both increases aqueous outflow and decreases aqueous humor formation. Beta blockers lower IOP by blockage of the beta-2 receptors in the ciliary process. Carbonic anhydrase inhibitors (CAIs) also decrease the rate of aqueous humor formation. Hyperosmotic agents lower IOP by increasing plasma tonicity, therefore drawing fluid out of the eye for rapid IOP decrease in the case of angle closure.

Lasers can be used to open the angle when medications fail to lower IOP. In open-angle glaucoma, the Argon laser is directed to the trabecular meshwork. Theoretically, this lowers the IOP when scar tissue forms, pulling the trabecular meshwork open. In angle closure glaucoma, a YAG laser iridotomy is used to create an opening in the iris. This allows the aqueous to pass through even if there is a pupillary block.

The goal in treating glaucoma is to control the IOP in order to eliminate, or at least minimize, damage to the patient's vision. Generally speaking, nerve damage (and, subsequently, lost vision) cannot be reversed by treatment.

For a complete understanding of glaucoma, glaucoma treatment, and tonometry, refer to the Basic Bookshelf Series titles, *Cataract and Glaucoma*, *Ocular Medications and Pharmacology*, and *Basic Procedures*.

Chapter 6

Uveal Tract, Pupil, and Anterior Chamber

KEY POINTS

- The iris can be a site of benign and malignant growths.

- A hypopyon is the accumulation of pus (white blood cells) in the anterior chamber. It may be caused by iritis, ulcers, keratitis, or trauma.

- A hyphema is a hemorrhage in the anterior chamber. It may occur spontaneously or result from trauma, iritis, neovascular glaucoma, or iridocyclitis.

- Uveitis is an inflammation of any of the uveal structures, including the iris, ciliary body, or choroid. Adjacent structures (such as the retina, vitreous, sclera, and cornea) are often secondarily involved.

Abnormalities/Disorders/Anomalies/Growths

Iris Growths

Iris cysts are rare, though often familial. Cysts in the peripheral portion of the iris may push directly over the trabecular meshwork, closing off the angle and causing angle-closure glaucoma. A gonioscope is usually required to see these cysts. When viewed with the gonioscope, the peripheral iris will have an unusually irregular contour. The cysts may sometimes be ruptured by performing an iridectomy using laser.

An iris leiomyoma is a lesion, resembling a melanoma, that is characterized by closely packed bundles of long spindle-shaped cells. It is a lightly pigmented yellowish, benign tumor which grows slowly. They are often removed as a precautionary measure.

Malignant melanomas of the iris are rare, and most arise from a preexisting nevus (which probably appeared unchanged for many years and then suddenly increased in size and became vascular). Advanced growth may spread into the ciliary body and block the angle of the anterior chamber, causing glaucoma. In the early stages, it may be possible to excise the sector of the iris containing the tumor, but when advanced it is necessary to enucleate the eye. The prognosis depends on the depth of the invasion. Malignant melanomas are usually metastatic from another part of the body and can be life-threatening.

Iris Freckles

Pigment flecks (iris freckles) are very common and are usually of no importance (Figure 6-1). Sometimes a larger nevus may grow and undergo malignant changes; therefore, it is important to have them observed periodically for changes.

Iris Coloboma

Iris coloboma is a fissure defect where the circle of the iris does not close completely during the time when the fetus is forming. Coloboma can range in severity from a small notch in the pupillary margin to an iris defect involving half or more of the iris. They usually occur in the inferior portion of the iris.

Iris Synechiea

Synechiea occur when a portion of the iris adheres to over- or under-lying structures. Anterior synechiea are adhesions of the iris to the corneal endothelium. Posterior synechiea occur between the iris and the lens. Such an adhesion can cause an abnormal pupil shape. They occur as a response to inflammation such as iritis or uveitis. If the adhesions impede the outflow of aqueous, a secondary angle-closure glaucoma may develop. The pupil is often dilated with eye drops in an attempt to break the adhesion(s).

Narrow Angle Structure

There is strong evidence to indicate that an abnormally narrow angle structure may be genetic. This defect usually causes no problems during childhood or young adulthood. In later life, however, a narrow angle may precipitate elevated IOP and/or attacks of angle-closure glaucoma. This

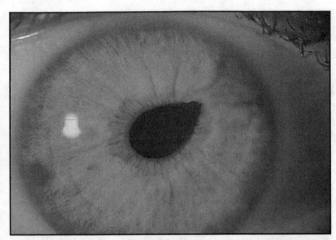

Figure 6-1. Iris nevi (Photograph by John Carswell).

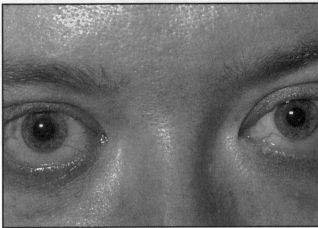

Figure 6-2. Anisocoria (Photograph courtesy of Todd Hostetter, COMT, CRA, FCLSA).

seems to occur slightly more often in men than women. Symptoms of elevated IOP are slight or absent in the early stages. An early diagnosis is of great importance to avoid permanent visual damage. Every person should have a complete eye examination (which should include tonometry and dilation) by age 40.

Anisocoria

OphA

Usually pupil size is the same in both eyes. Anisocoria refers to the unequal size of a patient's pupils, usually with a difference of one millimeter or more (Figure 6-2). About 25% of the normal population will have some degree of anisocoria from time to time. It may be caused by genetic defect, accident, medication, or chemicals. Pharmacologic testing to rule out Horner's Syndrome should be done.

Horner's Syndrome

OphA

Horner's Syndrome is a pathologic condition involving pupils, eyelids, and blood vessels of the facial skin. It is caused by damage to the third cranial (facial) nerve, which results in exposure of the inferior portion of the cornea. The affected side will exhibit decreased facial sweating (anhydrosis), lid droop (ptosis), and pupillary constriction (miosis) (Figure 6-3).

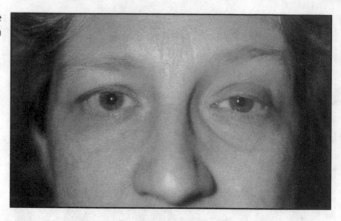

Figure 6-3. Horner's Syndrome (anisocoria OS > OD) (Photograph by John Carswell).

Pharmacological testing should be done to differentiate Horner's Syndrome from anisocoria. Accepted tests are done with cocaine, hydroxyamphetamine, or simple dilation drops.

The cocaine test involves instilling 5-10% ophthalmic cocaine in either eye. The dose is repeated 1 minute later. Horner's Syndrome is indicated by a pupil that dilates poorly to cocaine.

The cocaine test only tells us whether or not there is a Horner's Syndrome. The drug hydroxyamphetamine can separate a third-neuron Horner's Syndrome from first- and second-neuron syndromes. Hydroxyamphetamine 1% ophthalmic drops release packets of norepinephrine into the synaptic cleft (space between nerve cells). If the first or second neurons of the oculosympathetic system have been damaged and the final common pathway is intact, the third-order neurons are able to produce, transport, and store norepinephrine. Pupils dilate when Paredrine is instilled because norepinephrine is released. When the third-order neuron is damaged, there is no production, transport, or storage of norepinephrine. When Paredrine is instilled in the affected eye, no pupil dilation occurs. There is no test that can differentiate a first- and second-neuron Horner's Syndrome.

Dilation lag is a simple observation that aids in the diagnosis of Horner's Syndrome. Compared to the unaffected side, the affected pupil will dilate slower in the dark. Since the pupillodilator muscle actively dilates the pupil in darkness, damage to the sympathetic nerve supply will result in only passive release of the sphincter rather than active dilation. In dilation lag, photographs are taken 5 and 15 seconds after turning out the lights, using a close-up lens and flash.

Argyll Robertson's Syndrome

Normal pupils should be equal in size, shape, reaction to light, and reaction to accommodation. There should also be a decrease in pupil size when exposed to light or on reading closely. Argyll Robertson's Syndrome is a condition in which there is a failure of the direct and consensual light response of the pupil, but a normal reaction to accommodation. This abnormality is often due to a lesion in the midbrain light reflex path. It has been seen in diabetes mellitus, but neurosyphilis should be presumed until proven otherwise. Thus, a standard syphilis test should be performed on patients with Argyll Robertson's pupils.

Tonic Pupil

Tonic pupil (also known as Adie's tonic pupil) is the result of damage to the short posterior ciliary nerves. The pupil reacts poorly to light, but retains a reaction to near accommodation (although the response to near is tonic). When the patient looks at near and then refixates at distance, the pupil redilates very slowly.

Adie's pupil can be diagnosed by instilling 2.5% methacholine into the affected eye. This will constrict a tonic pupil, but will not affect a normal pupil.

Marcus Gunn Pupil

Marcus Gunn pupil, or afferent pupillary defect, is a diminished pupil reaction to light. It is usually caused by slowed conduction in the optic nerve fibers due to optic nerve disease. Its presence provides evidence of impaired function of the retina or optic nerve. The affected eye usually has poorer vision.

Consider an example in which the left eye has an afferent pupillary defect. If you shine a light into the normal right eye, both pupils will constrict. If you then move the light rapidly to the abnormal left eye, both pupils will dilate. This dilation may be barely noticeable or very dramatic. (The reaction is often graded on a scale of 1 to 4, with 4 being the most noticeable dilation.) Finally, if you move the light rapidly back to the right eye, pupillary constriction will again occur.

Note that the pupils do the same thing at the same time. This is because the innervation to the iridis respond to light equally. This phenomenon makes it possible to detect an afferent pupillary defect even if the affected eye has a fixed pupil. Again, suppose that the left eye has an afferent pupillary defect, but the pupil is non-reactive. When you shine the light in the right eye, the right pupil constricts. When you rapidly move the light to the left eye, the left pupil does not react, but the right pupil dilates. Finally, when you move the light back to the right eye, the right pupil will react with a rapid constriction (further evidence that it had dilated when the light was on the left eye).

Infections/Inflammations

Hypopyon

Hypopyon is the accumulation of pus (white blood cells) in the anterior chamber (Figure 6-4). It appears as a pool in the inferior portion of the anterior chamber. Hypopyons may be caused by iritis, ulcers, or keratitis. Often trauma to the eye results in hypopyon.

Hypopyons may be infective or sterile. They may be seen with a good light and the naked eye, but examination is best with a slit lamp examination.

Hyphema

A hyphema is a hemorrhage in the anterior chamber (Figure 6-5). It may be mild, with only red blood cells floating in the aqueous, or severe with the entire anterior chamber filling with blood (termed an 8-ball hyphema). A hyphema usually results from trauma to the globe. Other possible causes are iritis, neovascular glaucoma, iridocyclitis, and tumors. They sometimes occur spontaneously.

Decreased vision usually accompanies a hyphema. They usually resolve on their own. Hyphemas are viewed best with the slit lamp. The patient's IOP must be monitored, as blood cells may block the trabecular meshwork and impede the outflow of aqueous.

Uveitis

Uveitis is an inflammation of any of the structures of the uveal tract. This might include the iris and/or ciliary body in anterior uveitis, and the choroid in posterior uveitis. Although uveitis

Figure 6-4. Hypopyon (Photograph by Val Sanders, COT, CRA) (Reprinted from Ledford JK, Sanders VN. *The Slit Lamp Primer.* Thorofare, NJ: SLACK Incorporated; 1998).

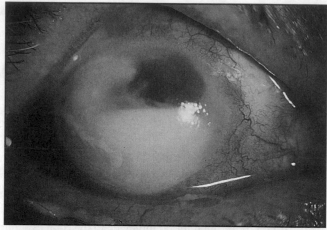

Figure 6-5. Hyphema (Photograph by Val Sanders, COT, CRA)

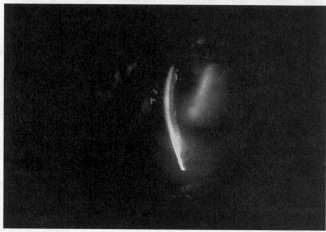

refers primarily to inflammation of this tract, adjacent structures such as the retina, vitreous, sclera, and cornea are also frequently involved.

Uveitis afflicts 2.3 million Americans (generally between the ages of 20 and 50) and causes 10% of all blindness. Of these patients, 75% have anterior uveitis (iritis, iridocyclitis).

Ocular signs and symptoms of iritis include tearing, blurred vision, miosis, pain, and redness. The patient's temperature may also be elevated.

Complications of iritis can be involvement of the cornea or sclera, secondary glaucoma, cataract, fundus changes, and acute angle-closure glaucoma.

Uveitis may occur in one eye or both. One single attack may occur, or the patient may have repeated episodes. An assortment of systemic infections and diseases may contribute to uveitis. Diseases that may contribute to anterior uveitis include Herpes simplex, Herpes zoster, Reiter's disease, and tuberculosis. Disorders that may be associated with posterior uveitis include histoplasmosis, toxoplasmosis, sarcoidosis, syphilis, toxocariasis, candidiasis, Lyme disease, sympathetic ophthalmia, and viral infections such as Herpes simplex and Herpes zoster, rubella, and rubeola.

Acute anterior uveitis usually has a sudden onset and lasts from 2 to 6 weeks. The pupil is constricted, and cells and flare are found in the anterior chamber. The patient has hyperemia, pain, photophobia, and blurred vision. In chronic anterior uveitis, these symptoms are not as severe.

OphA

Intermediate uveitis (pars planitis) is usually bilateral and often associated with multiple sclerosis. Patients present with blurred vision (from macula edema), floaters, and little or no pain. The ora serrata acquires a "snowbank" appearance inferiorly due to leakage from the tissues.

Posterior uveitis is limited entirely to the posterior segment of the eye. It is associated with little or no pain, minimum photophobia, minimum blurred vision (unless the macula is involved), and no perilimbal flush. Because of the anatomic closeness of the choroid and the retina, retinitis is usually present as well. If the macula is not involved, central vision may return to normal once the episode resolves.

Diagnosing uveitis requires analyzing the presence of an inflammation, a tumor, a vascular process, or a degeneration. The etiology of a uveitis is often unknown. Possible treatments include corticosteroids, mydriatic-cycloplegics, immunosuppressive drugs, nonsteroidal anti-inflammatory agents (NSAIDs), and photocoagulation.

Complications from uveitis might include band-shaped keratopathy, cataracts, macular surface wrinkling, edema of the disk and macula, corneal edema, and secondary glaucoma.

Crystalline Lens Overview

- The function of the lens is to focus incoming light onto the retina.

- In childhood and early adulthood, the lens is able to change shape in order to focus at close range (accommodation).

- The ability to accommodate is lost as we age (presbyopia), typically noticed by age 40.

- A cataract is an opacity in the crystalline lens. It is not a growth.

- A cataract can occur at any age, and in any part of the lens.

- The most common cause of cataracts is age. Other causes include heredity, long term steroid use, diabetes, injury, and exposure to radiation.

- Ninety-five percent of the population over age 65 has cataracts of various degrees of maturity.

- In the United States alone, over 1 million cataract extractions are performed each year.

Disorders of Lens Location

The crystalline lens is a focusing structure with an outer layer of epithelium covering concentric layers of fibers. The nucleus, the innermost part of the lens, contains the oldest cells. The crystalline lens is suspended by zonules from the ciliary process between the iris (anteriorly) and the vitreous humor (posteriorly). Lens position abnormalities involve luxation (total dislocation) and subluxation (partial dislocation).

Homocystinuria, a congenital abnormality involving dislocation of the lens, is an inherited autosomal recessive condition associated with an enzyme deficiency. Besides the subluxed lens, patients often have myopia, retinal detachment, glaucoma, and optic atrophy. Dislocation is usually bilateral and inferior. Patients frequently are developmentally delayed and suffer from osteoporosis. Special care must be taken if the patient requires ocular surgery with general anesthesia because of the frequency of arterial and venous thromboses. Other complications can include vitreous loss, iris prolapse, and retinal detachment.

In Marfan's syndrome, dislocation of the lens is usually upward. Marfan's syndrome is also inherited as autosomal dominant. Patients exhibit skeletal abnormalities, including a tall and thin body, scoliosis, and hyperextensible joints. They have normal intelligence. No chemical abnormality has been identified with Marfan's syndrome.

Ocular conditions associated with lens dislocations and/or detachments include aniridia, enlarged cornea, high myopia, intraocular tumor, and chronic uveitis.

The lens can be forcefully dislocated or detached due to trauma. Subtle dislocations that are not evident through the undilated pupil will likely manifest as a change in the patient's vision and refractive error. If the subluxed lens is sufficiently detached, iridodonesis (shaking of the iris) can be seen with a penlight.

A totally detached lens may float through the pupil and into the anterior chamber, where it may impede aqueous outflow and/or damage the corneal endothelium. Angle closure may also result if the luxated or subluxated lens moves forward to rest against the posterior face of the iris. A luxated lens that migrates into the posterior segment may cause a secondary open-angle glaucoma. Generally in these cases, the lens is surgically removed.

Presbyopia

The lens and the cornea form the optical system that ideally focuses light onto the retina. The crystalline lens changes shape to focus on closer objects (accommodation) when the ciliary muscle contracts and the zonular tension relaxes. This change reduces the focal length of the lens so that nearby objects are focused.

Infants possess great powers of accommodation. This power decreases with age as the lens lays down layers. The thickened, laminated lens is harder and not as flexible. By about age 40, much accommodative power has been lost (presbyopia) and reading glasses become necessary.

Cataracts

The nucleus of the lens changes and becomes increasingly yellow with age (nuclear sclerosis) due to compression as the lens thickens as well as other deteriorating and biochemical

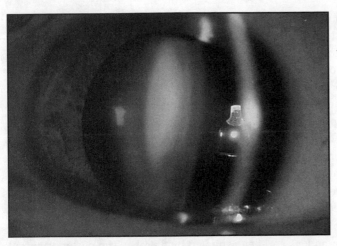

Figure 7-1. Cataract (Grade IV Nuclear Sclerosis) (Photograph by John Carswell).

changes. When the transparency of the crystalline lens decreases enough to disturb vision, a cataract exists (Figure 7-1). In addition, any lens opacity is termed a cataract.

Age is the most common cause of cataracts. Ninety-five percent of persons over age 65 have some degree of lens opacity. In the United States alone, over 1 million cataract extractions are performed each year. Cataracts account for 17 million cases of treatable blindness in the world. Surgery usually results in complete rehabilitation of vision.

The primary symptom of cataracts is decreased vision. Some patients describe this as a film or haze over their sight. Glare, distortion, halos around lights, decreased depth perception, and altered color perception may often become bothersome as well. Signs of cataract formation include a reduced visual acuity, and white or yellowish patches in the pupillary zone. Cataracts are best visualized through a dilated pupil with the slit lamp or ophthalmoscope.

Often cataracts mature quickly because of toxic effects from medications such as corticosteroids and miotics. Prolonged exposure to infrared radiation (glass blower, glass worker) can also lead to lens opacity. X-ray, microwave (radar installation workers), and ultraviolet (UV) radiation have also been associated with cataract formation. Additional risk factors include diabetes, smoking, extended use of steroids, over- or underweight, malnutrition, hypothyroid, and ocular trauma.

Cataracts can be classified according to the age at which they develop. The term "senile cataract" has been used to describe cataracts in older adults. Congenital cataracts are present at birth. Traumatic cataracts occur because of an injury.

Cataracts can also be classified by the area of the lens in which they occur. A cataract may be located in the center of the lens (nuclear cataract), on the posterior of the lens (posterior subcapsular), or in the peripheral cortex (cortical cataract).

The only treatment for cataracts of any type is surgical removal. Patients are generally recommended to have cataract extraction when vision decreases enough to compromise their daily visual needs. A thorough ophthalmologic evaluation, as well as a medical examination, is part of the normal preoperative course. Patients should have all the potential risks and medical complications completely explained to them. Surgery may be performed under local, topical, or general anesthesia. Most procedures are done in a certified outpatient facility. There is little disruption to the patient's normal living routine. (See Basic Bookshelf Series title *Overview of Ocular Surgery and Surgical Counseling*.)

Cataract extraction involves the total removal of the lens. Because the crystalline lens provides focusing power for the eye, this power is lost when the lens is extracted. In order to obtain

OptA

maximum vision, the aphakic eye (one without a crystalline lens) must be corrected by strong (+12.00) spectacle lenses, a contact lens, or an intraocular lens (IOL) implant. The IOL is the correction of choice, because it is placed inside the eye once the crystalline lens is removed during cataract surgery. An IOL is made of inert plastic, and can be placed in front of the iris (anterior IOL) or behind the pupil (posterior IOL).

Surgical techniques for cataract removal include intracapsular cataract extraction (ICCE), where the entire lens and intact capsule are removed. This procedure was widely used for nearly 50 years, but now has been almost entirely replaced by extracapsular cataract extraction (ECCE). ECCE removes the opaque portion of the lens without disturbing the posterior capsule or the anterior vitreous face. The posterior capsule serves as the site for the posterior chamber lens implant. Both ICCE and ECCE involve wound closure with several stitches. Generally, ECCE has fewer complications. The newest technique for cataract removal is phacoemulsification. This procedure involves liquifying the nucleus with a titanium needle which vibrates at ultrasonic frequencies. The pieces of the broken-up lens are then aspirated by a probe. The posterior capsule is left in place. Wound closure is accomplished with a single stitch or no stitch at all.

Sometimes the posterior capsule opacifies after cataract surgery. This is easily dealt with by creating an opening in the capsule itself. This is done on an outpatient basis using the infrared neodymium:yttrium-aluminum-garnet (Nd:YAG) laser.

For a more complete discussion of cataracts, see the Basic Bookshelf Series title *Cataract and Glaucoma*.

Chapter 8

Vitreous and Retina

KEY POINTS

- Vitreous floaters and detachments are generally benign conditions that are common among the middle-aged and elderly.

- Retinoblastoma is the most common childhood ocular malignancy. Leukocoria (white reflex in the pupil) is the most common presenting sign.

- Of patients between the ages of 20 and 74, diabetic retinopathy is the leading cause of new cases of blindness in the United States.

- Hypertension (high blood pressure) is estimated to affect some 15 million Americans. When elevated blood pressure is sustained, the arteries of the entire body (including the retina) are affected.

- Macular degeneration is the most common cause of vision loss in patients over 50 in the United States.

Abnormalities/Disorders/Anomalies/Growths

Floaters

Floaters are particles that are suspended in the vitreous. These particles cast shadows on the retina and are seen by the patient as spots. Those coming into the patient's line of vision are seen best against a plain background. Often floaters eventually settle below the line of sight.

Floaters normally occur with the aging process as the vitreous gel becomes more liquefied. Although floaters themselves are usually innocuous, they are occasionally indicative of more serious problems within the eye, such as iridocyclitis, retinal tears, vitreous hemorrhage, vitreous or retinal detachment, or inflammation.

Although rare, severe nonresolving vitreous opacities (eg, diabetic hemorrhage) require a vitrectomy, a surgical procedure which removes the vitreous, taking the opacities at the same time.

Asteroid Hyalosis

Asteroid hyalosis (also known as Benson's Disease) is a degenerative condition of the vitreous. Tiny, opaque, oval-shaped calcium deposits are found suspended in an essentially normal vitreous (Figure 8-1). These can be viewed with the slit lamp or ophthalmoscope. Asteroid hyalosis usually occurs in the elderly. In most cases, it is unilateral and causes no visual compromise.

Vitreous Detachment

Vitreous detachment is an innocuous condition that commonly occurs in middle-aged and elderly people. In youth, the vitreous is jelly-like. But as we age, the vitreous becomes more liquid-like, and may pull away from the underlying retina. As the vitreous tugs on the retina, light flashes occur. Patients often notice these light flashes in a dimly lit room. A shower of floaters may also accompany a vitreous detachment (also called posterior vitreous detachment, or PVD). Disease or trauma may also precipitate a PVD. Although a PVD itself is not visually threatening, the retina may tear at the point where the vitreous is tugging on it. In addition, the symptoms of PVD and retinal detachment are very similar. Therefore, any patient complaining of light flashes and floaters should be examined as soon as possible. Vitrectomy is the most significant advance in surgical management of vitreous detachment.

Retinoblastoma

Retinoblastoma is a retinal tumor that usually looks like a smooth, pink, rounded mass which may be single or multi-lobed. It may grow in or under the retina. The tumor may seep into the vitreous and grow back into the optic nerve. It may also extend into the anterior segment. If untreated, secondary tumors develop and gradually fill the eye, extending along the optic nerve to the brain, and end in death. Retinoblastoma is the most common childhood ocular malignancy. Of all cases of retinoblastoma, 60% are non-hereditary and 40% are hereditary. The most common presenting sign is a white reflex in the pupil. Strabismus is the second most common sign.

Treatment with radiation therapy is indicated if it is thought that the eye can be saved. If not, enucleation is the treatment of choice.

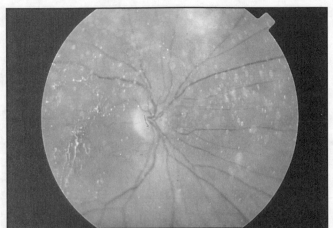

Figure 8-1. Asteroid hyalosis (Photograph by Val Sanders, COT, CRA).

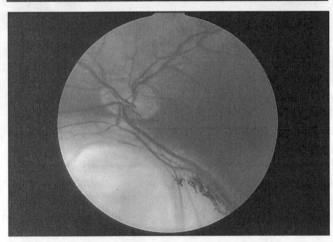

Figure 8-2. Retinal coloboma (Photograph courtesy of Todd Hostetter, COMT, CRA, FCLSA).

Retinal Coloboma

A retinal coloboma is a defect of the optic disc, usually manifested by the absence of the lower segment of the nerve head (Figure 8-2). It is caused by improper fusion of fetal fissure during gestation. Sixty percent of retinal colobomas occur bilaterally and are usually inherited.

Because all visual information generated by the retina must pass through the optic nerve, abnormalities of the optic nerve have serious visual effects. Retinal colobomas are usually associated with detachments of the macula late in life.

Diabetic Retinopathy

There are two types of diabetes. Type I (juvenile onset) diabetes cases are autoimmune. Type II (adult onset) has normal to high insulin production but insulin-resistant receptor cells. Type II diabetes is more prevalent than Type I.

Diabetes most often affects the retina, although it can affect the eye in many ways. As the disease advances, the retinal capillaries begin to deteriorate. This results in leakage of blood (hemorrhages) and fat-filled cells (exudates) into the retinal tissues. The retinal veins dilate because the capillaries are no longer able to carry oxygen and nutrients to the retina. This leads to areas of tissue death in the nerve fiber layer (cotton-wool spots). In an attempt to keep the tissues alive, new retinal blood vessels begin to sprout. This process is called neovascularization. Unfortunate-

Figure 8-3. Diabetic Retinopathy (Photograph courtesy of Todd Hostetter, COMT, CRA, FCLSA).

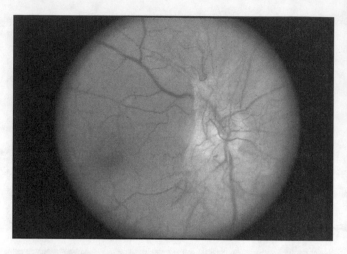

ly, the new vessels are abnormal and weak, and bleed easily. This results in more hemorrhages. The abnormal vessels also may grow into the macula.

Tissue death, exudates, infarcts, and neovascularization can each cause decreased vision. This entire scenario is collectively termed diabetic retinopathy (Figure 8-3). Of patients between the ages of 20 and 74, diabetic retinopathy is the leading cause of new cases of blindness in the United States. In diabetic retinopathy, the duration of insulin-dependency is the main contributing factor. In addition, Type I carries a higher risk of developing retinopathy.

Diabetic retinopathy is generally classified into two groups—background and proliferative. Background diabetic retinopathy (BDR) is distinguished by microaneurysms, hemorrhages, cotton-wool spots, exudates, intraretinal shunt vessels, and venous bleeding. The last two lesions (shunt vessels and venous bleeding) are sometimes referred to as a third classification, preproliferative retinopathy. Proliferative diabetic retinopathy (PDR) has abnormalities in the vessels on the surface of the retina or in the vitreous cavity. Neovascularization occurs at this stage. Vitreous hemorrhages and traction retinal detachments may also occur.

Because the retinal tissues and blood vessels are involved, fluorescein angiography and color fundus photography are used in the management of diabetic retinopathy. Good diabetic control and regular rechecks are required for patient care.

In severe cases, laser photocoagulation is done to achieve regression of existing vessels and inhibition of new vessel growth. Treating the entire retina with laser is done in stages. Focal laser treats just one specific area, and is used to seal off bleeding blood vessels.

Hypertensive Retinopathy

Hypertension (high blood pressure) is estimated to affect some 15 million Americans. When elevated blood pressure is sustained, the arteries of the entire body (including the retina) are affected and can cause death of the smooth muscle of the blood vessels. Blood plasma may then leak through the weakened, damaged vessel. (If fluorescein angiography is performed at this stage, this seepage appears as a leak of fluorescein.)

Retinal changes in patients with hypertensive retinopathy are classified into four groups. Group I exhibits abnormally narrowed and straightened blood vessels. The vessels may take on a brightened copper-silver reflex. These patients have "benign" hypertension, with no cardiac or renal dysfunction. In Group II patients, the vessels begin to leak. Small deposits and hemorrhages

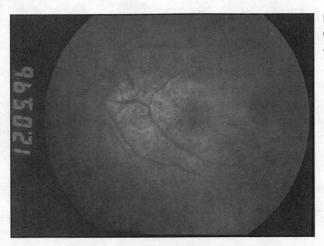

Figure 8-4. Age-related macular degeneration (Photograph by Angie Kasal, COT, OP).

may be evident. These patients are still in good health, but their blood pressure tends to run consistently high. Retinal changes in Group III include retinal edema, hemorrhages, and cotton-wool spots around the disk. A branch retinal vein occlusion may occur. Small areas of the retina may lose their blood supply, resulting in white patches of dead tissue (cotton-wool spots). These findings also occur in Group IV, along with disk edema. Patients in this group have the worst prognosis, because other organ systems (nervous system, kidneys, and other organs) have become affected as well.

Serious visual impairment usually does not occur as a result of hypertensive retinopathy unless there is local or venous occlusion. Because the blood vessels of the retina are involved, examination by ophthalmoscopy as well as fluorescein angiography are important. Patients with hypertension should have an annual eye exam that includes dilation.

The patient should have regular exams and blood pressure checks, as well as take his or her antihypertensive medication regularly. Retinopathy can often be reversed (especially in the early stages) if the blood pressure is adequately controlled with drugs. In some cases, retinal hemorrhages may be sealed with laser.

Macular Degeneration

Macular degeneration (also called age-related macular degeneration [ARMD] and senile macular degeneration [SMD]) is the most common cause of permanent vision loss in patients over 50 in the United States.

Macular degeneration is thought to occur when the retinal arteries become sclerosed. The lack of oxygen and nutrients causes the retinal tissue (primarily that of the macula) to break down (Figure 8-4). This results in a loss of central vision. Patients with macular degeneration complain of an inability to see to read, but most retain their peripheral vision, enabling them to "get around."

There are two types of age-related macular degeneration, dry and wet. Dry ARMD is less severe and visual loss progresses more slowly. In wet ARMD, new blood vessels have formed to try to cover the lack of oxygen to the tissues. These new vessels are weak, and tend to bleed and leak. This fluid can cause distortion and blurring of the central vision. The macula may actually detach. Wet ARMD is the cause of 90% of the cases of severe visual loss.

Because the central vision is affected, patients are often monitored by using an Amsler grid.

LV

OptA
OphA

The patient is to look at the grid (at home) every few days, and is instructed to contact the physician if any new change is noticed. The grid may also be used in the office to create a record of central vision changes.

Fluorescein angiography is also used in following macular degeneration, especially the wet type. Areas of low blood flow or leakage can be detected, and locations that might be treated with laser can be identified.

Patients with dry ARMD are generally advised to use stronger reading aids and low-vision aids. Some physicians advocate vitamin therapy, especially Vitamins A, C, E, and zinc. Alternately, there are many "ocular" vitamins now on the market. Wet ARMD can sometimes be treated with laser, but this is decided on a case-by-case basis because of the risks of applying laser too close to the macula. Since vision that has already been lost cannot be restored, treatment is aimed at preventing further loss.

Retinal and Macular Holes

Because the macula is the area of central vision, if a hole occurs in the macula the visual results can be devastating. Visual distortion may also occur if there is accompanying macular edema. While a macular hole can happen at any age, it is more common in the elderly (especially women in the 60 to 70 year bracket.) The patient and the eye are often otherwise healthy. The cause of most macular holes is unknown, and it may be partial or full thickness (Figure 8-5). No treatment can restore vision or close the hole. If a retinal detachment occurs, treatment is undertaken to preserve the rest of the retina (see Retinal Detachment, below).

Retinal holes can occur in the periphery of the retina. They are often associated with retinopathy of prematurity. For their detection, an indirect ophthalmoscope is needed (along with a fully-dilated pupil). In the adult, fluorescein angiography may also be used.

Retinal Detachment

In retinal detachment (RD), the retina separates from the underlying retinal pigment epithelium (Figure 8-6). Fluid gets under the retinal layers, causing a fluid wedge between the two. This fluid may come from the vitreous, which gains access between the layers through a retinal hole or tear. This is known as a rhegmatogenous RD, which is the most common type of RD. Or, blood or plasma may exude from blood vessels in the choroid or retina, pushing the layers apart. This is a secondary (or serous and hemorrhagic) RD. Finally, fibrous bands in the vitreous (which are attached to the retina) may retract and pull the retina away from its base. This is a traction RD.

Symptoms of RD may include light flashes, floaters, some loss of vision, a veil or curtain before the eyes, or no symptoms at all. The retina will appear gray and opaque, rather than its usual pink color. The retina may be examined via ophthalmoscope or ultrasound.

The rhegmatogenous type of RD is often associated with trauma, aphakia, and myopia (usually of 6.00 diopters or greater). A posterior vitreous detachment may precede the detachment of the retina in any of these cases. The secondary type of RD is often seen in disorders involving degeneration or inflammation, as well as any disorder where neovascularization has occurred. Traction retinal detachment occurs most often in long-term diabetics, but may also be related to trauma or prematurity. For more details see the Basic Bookshelf Series title, *Ocular Emergencies*.

A retinal detachment requires immediate repair. This may be undertaken via scleral buckling,

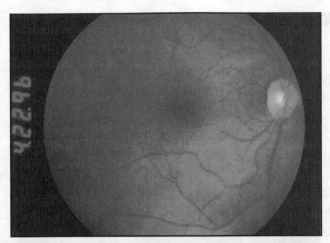

Figure 8-5. Macular hole (Photograph by Angie Kasal, COT, OP).

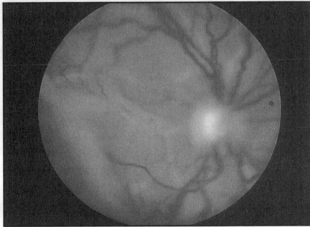

Figure 8-6. Retinal detachment (Photograph courtesy of Todd Hostetter, COMT, CRA, FCLSA).

pneumatic retinopexy, cryotherapy, diathermy, or laser. Surgical reattachment is reported to be successful about 90% of the time.

Retinopathy of Prematurity

Retinopathy of Prematurity (ROP) is, as its name implies, a retinal disorder affecting individuals who were born before term. (The term retrolental fibroplasia is a term that was used for awhile to refer to ROP, but has now fallen out of use.) The disorder was first believed to be caused by the administration of oxygen to premature newborns. However, it is now believed that prematurity itself, with its associated low birth weight, is the actual cause. Medical advances have made it possible to save smaller and smaller "preemies," however, it is these smallest babies who are at the highest risk for developing ROP.

The scenario of ROP includes retinal neovascularization, dilated and twisted retinal blood vessels, and peripheral retinal detachment. About 500 babies born in the United States each year will be blind due to ROP. However, many infants undergo a regression of retinopathy by the 15th week of life. Even in regression there may be side effects of ROP. These can include a stretched macula, myopia, strabismus, cataract, and angle-closure glaucoma. In severe, unregressed cases, treatment may include cryotherapy, laser and vitreoretinal surgery.

LV

Figure 8-7. Choroidal nevus (Photograph by Angie Kasal, COT, OP).

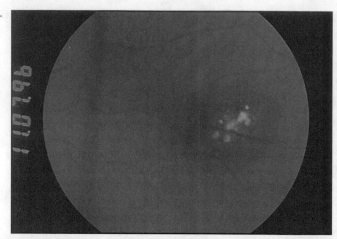

Figure 8-8. Retinitis (Photograph courtesy of Todd Hostetter, COMT, CRA, FCLSA).

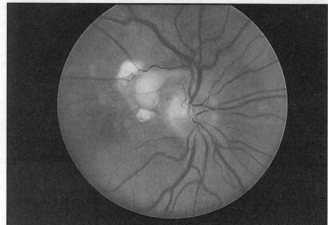

Choroidal Nevus

A choroidal nevus is a benign lesion located in the blood vessel layer of the choroid (Figure 8-7). It may be a pigmented or non-pigmented freckle that causes no harm; however, it can be difficult to tell a nevus from a malignant melanoma. Patients with choroidal nevi should be monitored regularly. Typically, a nevus does not grow and remains flat.

Infections/Inflammations

Retinitis

The term retinitis refers to any inflammation of the retina (Figure 8-8). Pure retinitis (in which only the retina is involved) is rare, however. Usually there is also involvement of the choroid and vitreous. Retinochoroiditis, chorioretinitis, and endophthalmitis are all used to describe inflammatory changes in the inner eye which may include retinal inflammation. The cause of retinitis is usually infective, due to bacteria, viruses (including Herpes), or fungi (most commonly *Candida*). Patients who are immunocompromised are especially at risk.

A vascular response of the involved tissue is the most visible change seen in an inflammatory process that includes the retina. Inflammatory cells spill into the retinal tissue and accumulate around the blood vessels. These cells appear as white opacities. Migration of the cells into the vitreous causes floaters and vitreous haze. Hemorrhages may occur in the retina and, occasionally, in the vitreous. The retinal response may also include folding and scarring. There is usually a loss of central vision because the macula is directly involved, or there is retinal edema or detachment. Treatment depends on the causative agent, but may include antibiotics or pars plana vitrectomy.

Vitritis

Vitritis refers to inflammation of the vitreous. In most cases, inflammatory products from the posterior segment of the eye have spilled over into the vitreous. The vitreous responds by liquification, opacification, and shrinkage whenever it is exposed to an inflammatory process. Inflammatory products within the vitreous body can induce organization of fibrous membranes. These fibers may pull on the retina, causing traction retinal detachments. Vitritis may be associated with posterior uveitis, tuberculosis, toxoplasmosis, and syphilis. If the posterior segment is inflamed due to bacterial infection, the vitreous may become involved as well, leading to endophthalmitis. (The vitreous is an excellent culture medium for the growth of bacteria.)

Chapter 9

Optic Nerve

KEY POINTS

- The physiologic cup is the area in the middle of the optic disc; it is a slightly reddish depression which appears in the normal eye.

- Research has indicated that patients with large, round cups and a cup-to-disc ratio exceeding 0.6 (ie, 60%) are more at risk for developing glaucoma.

- Optic nerve atrophy is a degeneration of the nerve fibers, causing decreased vision.

- Optic neuritis is an inflammation of the optic nerve which usually causes a slow, progressive loss in visual acuity.

Abnormalities/Disorders/Anomalies/Growths

Optic Disc Cupping

The normal, healthy optic nerve head (disc) has a small depression in its center, known as the physiologic cup. The cup appears slightly reddish when compared to the whiteness of the rest of the disc. The size of the cup varies from one individual to another, but the shape of a normal cup is generally round.

In glaucoma, however, the increased intraocular pressure (IOP) can begin to "excavate" the normal cup. Optic disc cupping refers to an abnormal increase in the size of the physiologic cup. The shape of an abnormal cup is generally more oval in the vertical directions (typically progressing toward the inferior pole of the disc first, and then superiorly). As cupping increases, the nerve fibers are damaged. This causes a loss in the peripheral visual fields. Defects manifest in opposite positions than they are anatomically located. Thus, cupping close to the inferior pole of the disc will result in superior field loss, and cupping close to the superior pole will result in inferior field loss.

Because of the connection between elevated IOP and cupping, examination of the optic nerve head is key in the diagnosis and management of glaucoma. Cupping is documented by means of the cup-to-disc ratio. This ratio compares the diameter of the cup to the diameter of the disc. In the normal eye, the cup is usually no more than a third of the size of the disc. If the cup was 1/3 the size of the disc, this would be noted as .3 or a 30% cup. If the cup took up half the space of the disc, this would be called a .5 or 50% cup. In the late stages of glaucoma, if the cup occupied the entire disc space, we would say that the disc was "cupped out," or use a cup-to-disc ratio of 1.0 or 100%.

Research has indicated that patients with large, round cups and a cup-to-disc ratio exceeding 0.6 (ie, 60%) are more at risk for developing glaucoma. Large "normal" cups are usually round in shape, while discs of patients with glaucoma are elongated vertically, as indicated above. In addition, it is possible to find glaucomatous cupping in patients whose IOP is within normal range. If visual field loss has also occurred, these patients are said to have normal tension glaucoma, and are usually put on antiglaucoma medications. If visual field loss has not occurred, the patient might be diagnosed as a glaucoma suspect, and monitored carefully.

Optic Nerve Atrophy

Optic nerve atrophy is degeneration of the optic nerve fibers (Figure 9-1). If the nerve fibers deteriorate to the point of death, they cannot be regenerated. The patient may notice a loss in color perception and/or blind spots in the vision.

Optic nerve atrophy can be caused by a decrease in the nerve fiber count with advancing age or by medical conditions that accelerate the process, such as glaucoma. There is an hereditary type of optic atrophy that affects mainly males. Lyme disease, syphilis, drug reactions, and trauma often are causes of disease-related optic atrophy. A secondary optic atrophy may follow chronic papilledema or papillitis.

Optic atrophy is treated by treating the causative condition. The sooner treatment is initiated, the better the chances for recovery. Hereditary optic atrophy is not treatable, and vision loss is almost always permanent.

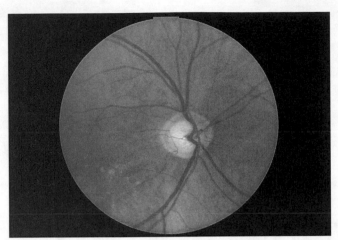

Figure 9-1. Optic nerve atrophy (Photograph courtesy of Todd Hostetter, COMT, CRA, FCLSA).

Infections/Inflammations

Optic Neuritis

Optic neuritis is an inflammation or degeneration of the optic nerve (Figure 9-2) commonly associated with multiple sclerosis (MS), Lyme disease, or neurosyphilis. It may also occur with infections from the meninges, orbital tissues, or paranasal sinuses. In some cases, the neuritis may be part of a drug reaction (notably chloramphenicol, streptomycin, sulfa drugs, Diabinese [Pfizer Inc, New York, NY], or birth control pills). However, in many cases, the cause is unknown. If a cause cannot be found, there is a 40% chance that the patient will develop MS within the next 2 years.

Optic neuritis usually occurs in only one eye, and the patient first complains of moderate to severe pain or soreness. Visual changes usually begin a day or two after the pain. Transient blurring may occur, with episodes that last from several minutes to several hours. Alternately, the vision may gradually decrease over a period of days. Color perception, depth perception, and peripheral vision may also be affected. Some patients note blind spots in the central or peripheral vision.

Optic neuritis may also be referred to as retrobulbar neuritis, papillitis, or neuroretinitis. Retrobulbar neuritis occurs far enough behind the optic nerve so that no abnormality is visible in the fundus. Papillitis refers to conditions in which the disc is swollen and hyperemic. (Some experts use "papillitis" as a broad heading, under which they include optic neuritis and ischemic optic neuropathy). Neuroretinitis is the same as papillitis except that the process has moved out into the adjacent retinal and uveal tissues.

If MS is the cause, treatment involves oral or intravenous steroids. Otherwise, the patient will probably not receive any treatment and the disorder is allowed to run its course. Prognosis for a full visual recovery is guarded, even though 75% of the cases show some improvement in visual acuity. Recovery may take 7 months to over a year.

Papilledema

Papilledema (also referred to as a "choked disc") is swelling of the optic nerve not caused by inflammation, but rather by increased intracranial pressure. This pressure may be caused by a

Figure 9-2. Optic neuritis (Photograph courtesy of Todd Hostetter, COMT, CRA, FCLSA).

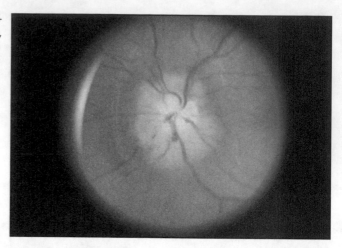

head injury or infection. It has also been associated with rheumatic or congenital heart disease. The elevated intracranial pressure squeezes the optic nerve, preventing transmission along the nerve fibers. In addition, the pressure may force fluid into the nerve, further increasing the pressure. The patient may notice 1-minute episodes of blurred vision, with normal vision after each attack. Double vision, decreased side vision, and headaches may also occur. The problems may occur in one eye or both.

If optic atrophy already exists, papilledema cannot occur. Long-standing papilledema may cause optic atrophy.

Papilledema is considered a medical emergency, and the patient is usually hospitalized at once. Treatment is aimed at lowering the intracranial pressure. A spinal tap may be done to remove fluid and thus lower the pressure. Diuretics may also be used to reduce the overall amount of fluid in the body. If an infection is associated with the papilledema, the infection should be treated. Once the intracranial pressure is normalized, vision recovers over a 6- to 8-week period.

Ischemic Optic Neuropathy

Ischemic optic neuropathy (ION) occurs when there is nerve tissue degeneration due to blocked arteries in the optic nerve. When the blood supply to the optic nerve is cut off, tissue deterioration begins because the nerve fibers have no source of oxygen. ION is often associated with temporal arteritis, hypertension, diabetes, and hypercholesterolemia. The patient may experience a sudden vision loss, or there may be episodes of transient vision loss prior to the major loss. In some cases the patient may notice blind spots in the periphery. The condition is usually painless, although some patients complain of a temporal headache. The pupil in the affected eye may be larger or exhibit a pupillary defect. If only one eye is affected, it is likely that the other eye will become affected later (within a few hours of the fellow eye, or even several years later).

Recovery varies with the cause of the disorder. Treatment usually includes oral steroids in a decreasing dose, sometimes over the course of several months. The causative disease will also be fully examined and treated if necessary.

Neurological Conditions

- Several of the cranial nerves are involved in visual function. Palsies of the third, fourth, and sixth nerves affect the extraocular muscles.

- Strabismus refers to the misalignment of eyes caused by extraocular muscle or nerve problems.

- Pupils should be inspected for size, shape, and reaction to direct and consensual light, as well as accommodative reflex.

Eye Movements

Eye movements are controlled by the extraocular muscles. The medial rectus (MR) causes the eye to turn inward (adduct) toward the nose. The lateral rectus (LR) causes the eye to turn outward (abduct) horizontally. The superior rectus (SR), the inferior rectus (IR), the superior oblique (SO), and the inferior oblique (IO) produce various combinations of vertical, horizontal, and rotary movements, depending on the position of the eyes.

Nystagmus

Nystagmus is a neurological disorder in which there are involuntary, rhythmic movements of one or both eyes. These movements might occur in one or all fields of gaze, and may be described as pendular or jerk movements. In pendular nystagmus, the movement of the eye in one direction is followed by an equal movement in the opposite direction. In jerk nystagmus, the initial motion is slow followed by a more rapid recovery movement. The extent to which the eye moves is referred to as the amplitude of the nystagmus. The rate of nystagmus is the frequency of the movements. In most cases, the smaller the amplitude, the faster the rate. The opposite also holds true. The movements may be horizontal, vertical, or cyclic.

There are nearly 40 documented types of nystagmus. The condition may be congenital or acquired; the acquired type is sometimes associated with visual dysfunction, drug reaction (notably to sedatives and anticonvulsants), or damage to the brain stem. Other disorders sometimes linked to nystagmus are multiple sclerosis, severe inner ear problems, alcoholism, stroke, and myasthenia gravis.

The patient with congenital nystagmus typically has decreased vision because the constant motion of the eyes creates a blur. Since there is never a clear image, the child frequently develops amblyopia. Often the movements decrease or stop in one position of gaze or another. The child unconsciously learns to tilt or turn the head in a specific direction in order to place the eyes in the quieter position. Nystagmus often increases if one eye is occluded. Because of this, use a high plus lens (+6.00, for example) as an occluder when performing refractometry. It might also be helpful to perform the refractive measurement using trial frames and allowing the patient to adopt the preferred head position.

A normal patient may exhibit nystagmus when the eyes are directed to extreme left or right gaze. This is known as end-point nystagmus, and is not considered pathologic. Optokinetic nystagmus, also a normal phenomenon, may also be elicited in a healthy individual by having him or her concentrate on passing repetitive targets such as the optokinetic drum or tape. (A more natural example is a passenger in a car watching fence posts pass by.)

Nerve Palsies

Several of the cranial nerves are involved with visual function. The third, fourth and sixth nerve affect extraocular muscle movement. A problem in the conduction of impulses along any of these nerves can thus affect muscle balance. A dysfunction of the seventh nerve affects lid closure.

Third nerve palsy (oculomotor nerve palsy) can affect the SR, IR, and MR, levator, and IO muscles. The pupil sphincter and ciliary muscles are affected as well. Typically the patient experiences double vision (usually horizontal) which may resolve if the head is turned to the left or right. Ptosis, an enlarged pupil, and cycloplegia (so that the patient might complain of poor near vision) occur on the affected side. The condition can develop rapidly, and may affect one or both eyes. Risk factors include diabetes, multiple sclerosis, hypertension, migraine, head injury, myasthenia gravis, recent viral infection (notably of the inner ear or sinus), inflammation, and aneurysm. The condition is not actually treated, although patching or prisms may be used to relieve the diplopia. Recovery, if it occurs, may take 6 months. If the condition persists, surgery may be recommended.

A fourth nerve palsy (trochlear nerve palsy) affects the superior oblique muscle. The patient generally experiences diagonal double vision, although the images may be vertical. The diplopia may resolve if the patient tilts his or her head toward one shoulder. Onset is usually sudden. Conditions implicated in a fourth nerve palsy include head injury (most common), multiple sclerosis, myasthenia gravis, tumor, and aneurysm. As with a third nerve palsy, the diplopia may be relieved with patching or prisms. If the condition has not resolved in 6 months, surgery may be considered.

Sixth nerve palsy (abducens nerve palsy) affects the lateral rectus muscle. Thus, the patient experiences horizontal diplopia, which may improve with a head turn to the right or left. Disorders associated with a sixth nerve palsy include hypertension, migraine, arteriosclerosis, head injury, recent viral infection (notably of the inner ear or sinuses), Lyme disease, tumor, and increased intracranial pressure. Patching, prisms, and observation are again the order of the day, with surgery considered in unresolved cases.

A seventh nerve palsy (Bell's palsy, facial palsy, facial nerve palsy) causes paralysis of the face so that there is no expression on that side. The palsy may be complete or partial. The patient may first notice pain behind the ear; facial paralysis follows within several hours. Because the seventh nerve controls the orbicularis muscle, a nerve palsy can render the eye unable to close. Thus, corneal drying is an urgent problem. The cause of the palsy is usually unknown, although it has occasionally been associated with dental procedures. Ocular lubricants throughout the day and taping the eye shut at night are usually recommended. If the paralysis is partial, recovery may occur over a period of months. If the paralysis is total, there may be resolution depending on what part of the nerve is involved.

Strabismus

Strabismus refers to the misalignment of eyes caused by an extraocular muscle or nerve problem. Because the eyes are not aligned, the image of an object falls on the fovea of one eye, but not the other. If the deviation is occurring for the first time in an adult (due to a nerve palsy, for example), the patient will have double vision. A child with strabismus learns to "turn off" the extra image and does not see double. If the same eye is continually "turned off," that eye will not learn to see optimally and amblyopia will develop.

Strabismus in which one eye is constantly out of alignment is called a tropia. (Actually, a tropia may be constant or intermittent.) In addition, there is latent strabismus which does not appear unless fusion is disrupted; this is known as a phoria. Whether a tropia or phoria, the direction of the deviation is important. If the eye turns out, this is an exo (exotropia or exophoria). An in-turned eye is said to be eso (esotropia or esophoria). If the eyes are misaligned vertically, we usually designate it by the higher eye as hyper (hypertropia; a vertical phoria is rare).

The primary position of gaze is the position assumed by the eyes when fixating on a distant object directly ahead. Secondary positions include the near-fixation position, the six cardinal positions, and the two midline positions. In comitant strabismus, the same degree of misalignment occurs in all directions of gaze and there is no ocular muscle paralysis. In noncomitant strabismus, an extraocular muscle is affected, which makes the misalignment different in various positions of gaze.

A complete explanation of strabismus is beyond the scope of this text, but is available in the Basic Bookshelf Series title, *A Systematic Approach to Strabismus*.

Pupils

Pupillary abnormalities are discussed in Chapter 6, although a few notes are presented here.

Normal pupils are equal in size, ranging from 3 to 5 mm in normal room light. Pupils tend to be larger in childhood and smaller in elderly people. Pupils smaller than 3 mm are miotic, which could be caused from certain drugs for glaucoma (such as pilocarpine) or using drugs such as heroin. Pupils larger than 7 mm are mydriatic, which may be caused from ocular contusion, systemic poisoning, or neurologic disease. Anisocoria is when the two pupils are not equal in size.

The pupils are normally round in shape. Irregularly shaped pupils that have not undergone surgical intervention may be affected by congenital abnormality (coloboma), syphilis, trauma, or "scarring down" from iritis.

Visual Fields

The purpose of visual field testing is to determine the outer limits of the visual perception and the qualities of vision within that area. Some disorders cause specific patterns of loss in the visual field. Interpretation of visual fields is therefore important in diagnosing disease and locating lesions in the visual pathway, as well as for following changes as diseases progress. Each eye is tested separately. The tested eye fixates on a central target, and the patient is asked to respond to lights or targets in the periphery. Sensitivity of the various areas of the visual field may be tested with lights of various size and intensity.

A complete review of visual fields is found in the Basic Bookshelf Series title, *Visual Fields*.

Bibliography

Abelson M, Parver L. How to treat uveitis. *Review of Ophthalmology*. August 1995; 107-110.

Abelson M, Welch D. How to treat bacterial conjunctivitis. *Review of Ophthalmology*. December 1994; 44-45.

Ai E, Ahmed I. How to handle CME (cystoid macula edema). *Review of Ophthalmology*. June 1996; 86-89.

Apple D, Rabb M. *Ocular Pathology—Clinical Applications and Self Assessments*. St. Louis, Mo: Mosby-Year Book, Inc; 1991.

Asbell P, Foulks G, Gilbard J, Richardson T, Tabor J. *Update on Dry Eye Syndromes—Guidelines on the Diagnosis and Management of Conditions Called "Dry Eye."* New Orleans, La: CLAO Monograph; 1996.

Basinger K, Johnson Y. No-nonsense solutions to the tear dilemma. *Spectrum*. April 1994; 20-24.

Berger B. How to manage iridocyclitis. *Review of Ophthalmology*. August 1995; 103-106.

Bergren R, Doft B. How to manage endophthalmitis. *Review of Ophthalmology*. June 1996; 74-84.

Bruce A, Brennan N. Corneal pathophysiology with contact lens wear. *Surv Ophthalmol*. 1990; 35(1): 25-51.

Caffery B. Proper lid hygiene can be a simple dry eye solution. *Spectrum*. June 1994; 49.

Campbell R, Caroline P. Mechanical trauma and GPC. *Spectrum*. September 1995; 56.

Campbell R, Caroline P. Meibomian gland dysfunction. *Spectrum*. November 1995; 56.

Cassin B, ed. *Fundamentals for Ophthalmic Technical Personnel*. Philadelphia, Pa: WB Saunders; 1995.

Cassin B, Solomon S. *Dictionary of Eye Terminology*. Gainesville, Fla: Triad Publishing Company; 1984.

Cavallerano A. Understanding acquired macular disorders and choroidal neovascularization. *Spectrum*. February 1994; 42-52.

Davis R. Corneal infiltrates: what are they all about? *Eye Quest Magazine*. June 1995; 14.

Donnenfeld E, Kanellopoulos A. When corneal disease threatens the globe. *Review of Ophthalmology*. August 1996; 48-56.

Dowey W. *What is Keratoconus?* Los Angeles, Calif: The National Keratoconus Foundation; 1995.

Duane T, et al. *Clinical Ophthalmology Series*. Hagerstown, Md: Harper & Roe; 1980.

Epstein Arthur, et al. Handling clinical complications. *Contact Lens Forum*. March 1991; 11-15.

Faherty B. Chronic blepharitis: easy nursing interventions for a common problem. *Journal of Ophthalmic Nursing and Technology*. 1992; 11(1): 20-22.

Fedukowiez H, Stenson S. *External Infections of the Eyes—Bacterial, Viral, Mycotic with Noninfectious and Immunologic Diseases*. Norwalk, Conn: Appleton-Century-Crofts; 1985.

Finnemore V. How the eyelids help and hurt contact lens wear. *Spectrum*. February 1994; 26-29.

Fisch B. Clinical management of eyelid disease. *Spectrum*. February 1991; 40-52.

Fisch B. Corneal ulcers and contact lens wear. *Spectrum*. May 1990; 48-58.

Friedlaender M, Bartlett J. Getting a handle on dry eye. *Eye Care Technology*. May 1996; 33-50.

Gasset A. *Contact Lenses and Corneal Disease*. New York, NY: Appleton-Century-Crofts; 1976.

Gayton JL, Ledford JR. *The Crystal Clear Guide to Sight for Life*. Lancaster, Pa: Starburst Publishers; 1996.

Gilbard J. New possibilities in managing dry eye patients. *Ophthalmology World News*. February 1995; 35-36.

Gilbard JP. *Principles and Practice of Ophthalmology*. Philadelphia, Pa: WB. Saunders Co; 1994.

Grohe R. A complete guide to detecting and managing limbal complications. *Spectrum*. June 1994; 26-29.

Gwin N, Anderson D. *Red Flags: Recognizing Contact Lens Complications*. Paper submitted at Contact Lens Society of America meeting, San Antonio, Tex; 1996.

Hannush S. What's new in cornea and external disease. *Review of Ophthalmology*. April 1996; 66-70.

Henkind P, Starida R. *Atlas of Glaucoma*. Fort Worth, Tex: Medical Dialogues, Inc; 1984.

Hood D. Do soft lens solutions cause corneal infiltrates? *Spectrum*. February 1994; 20-23.

Jennings B. Anterior uveitis - diagnosing and treating ocular inflammatory disease. *Eye Quest Magazine*. July/August 1996; 32-45.

Lacrisertä on-line product information. (No longer accessible.) http://www.rxmed.com/monographs/lacrisrt.htm/lacrisrt®

Larke J. *The Eye in Contact Lens Wear*. Great Britain: Butler and Tanner Ltd; 1985.

Lee F. Nutrition's role in age-related ocular disease. *Spectrum*. August 1995; 38-48.

Keratoconjunctivitis sicca or dry eye. http://www.netrover.com/-eyevet/kcs.html. Access date 8/7/96.

McNamara JA, Moreno R, Tasman WS. *Retinopathy of prematurity*. In: Tasman W, Jaeger EA, eds. Duane's Ophthalmology on CD-ROM. Philadelphia, PA: Lippincott-Raven Publishers; 1996.

Meisler D, Keller W. Contact lens type, material, and deposits and giant papillary conjunctivitis. *CLAO Journal*. 1995; 21(1): 77-80.

Miller D, White P. Infectious and inflammatory contact lens complications. *Spectrum*. May 1995; 40.

Newsome D, Khadem J, Weiter J. The role of vitamins in macular degeneration. *Review of Ophthalmology*. June 1996; 112-114.

Ong B. Clinical diagnosis and management of meibomian gland dysfunction. *Spectrum*. June 1996; 31-36.

Onofrey B, Lee M. Management of ocular surface disease. *Eye Quest Magazine*. June 1995; 36-47.

Paton D, Hyman BN, Justice J Jr. *Introduction to Ophthalmoscopy*. Kalamzaoo, Mich: Upjohn Co; 1976.

Pau H. *Differential Diagnosis of Eye Disease*. New York, NY: Thieme Medical Publishers, Inc; 1988.

Pavan-Langsten D. *Manual of Ocular Diagnosis and Therapy*. Boston, Mass: Little, Brown, and Company; 1996.

Redmond J. A different way to handle aqueous deficiency. August 1994. On-line source: http://www.revophth.com/rph4f6.htmatoconjunctivitis. Access date 1/2/97.

Rosenthal B, Faye E. Current concepts on macular degeneration. *Eye Quest Magazine*. May 1995; 36-48.

Scheid T. Microcysts and reversed illumination. *Spectrum*. June 1996; 39-40.

Schnider C. Fingerprint "dystrophy." *Spectrum*. June 1994; 19.

Smith R, Flowers C. Chronic blepharitis: a review. *CLAO Journal*. 1995; 21(3): 200-207.

Spencer W. *Ophthalmic Pathology—An Atlas and Textbook*. Philadelphia, Pa: WB Saunders Company; 1985.

Stein H, Slatt B. *The Ophthalmic Assistant*. St. Louis, Mo: The CV Mosby Company; 1983.

Townsend W. Medications for contact lens-related infection. *Spectrum*. May 1996; 41-48.

Vaughn D, Cook R, Asbury T. *General Ophthalmology*. Los Altos, Calif: Appleton & Lange; 1968.

Vaughan DG, Asbury T, Riordan-Eva P. *General Ophthalmology, 13th ed*. Norwalk, Conn: Appleton & Lange; 1992.

Vickery JA. *Contact Lens and the Dry Eye Patient*. Research paper presented as a private lecture; 1992.

Index

*F*or *your information*

This book and many others on numerous different topics are available from SLACK Incorporated. For further information or a copy of our latest catalog, contact us at:

Professional Book Division
SLACK Incorporated
6900 Grove Road
Thorofare, NJ 08086 USA
Telephone: 1-609-848-1000
1-800-257-8290
Fax: 1-609-853-5991
E-mail: orders@slackinc.com
WWW: http://www.slackinc.com

We accept most major credit cards and checks or money orders in US dollars drawn on a US bank. Most orders are shipped within 72 hours.

Contact us for information on recent releases, forthcoming titles, and bestsellers. If you have a comment about this title or see a need for a new book, direct your correspondence to the Editorial Director at the above address.

*If you are an instructor, we can be reached at the address listed above or on the Internet at **educomps@slackinc.com** for specific needs.*

Thank you for your interest and we hope you found this work beneficial.